D0489390

teach
yourself

Books are to be returned on or before
the last date below.

massage

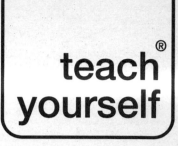

massage
denise whichello brown
B.Sc., Cert. Ed., D.O., M.A.O.

For over 60 years, more than
40 million people have learnt over
750 subjects the **teach yourself**
way, with impressive results.

be where you want to be
with **teach yourself**

For UK order enquiries: please contact Bookpoint Ltd., 130 Milton Park, Abingdon, Oxon OX14 4SB. Telephone: +44 (0) 1235 827720. Fax: +44 (0) 1235 400454. Lines are open from 09.00–18.00, Monday to Saturday, with a 24-hour message answering service. You can also order through our website www.madaboutbooks.com

For USA order enquiries: please contact McGraw-Hill Customer Services, PO Box 545, Blacklick, OH 43004-0545, USA. Telephone: 1-800-722-4726. Fax: 1-614-755-5645.

For Canada order enquiries: please contact McGraw-Hill Ryerson Ltd., 300 Water St, Whitby, Ontario L1N 9B6, Canada. Telephone: 905 430 5000. Fax: 905 430 5020.

Long-renowned as the authoritative source for self-guided learning – with more than 30 million copies sold worldwide – the *Teach Yourself* series includes over 300 titles in the fields of languages, crafts, hobbies, business, computing and education.

British Library Cataloguing in Publication Data: A catalogue record for this title is available from The British Library.
Library of Congress Catalog Card Number: on file

First published in UK 1996 by Hodder Headline Ltd., 338 Euston Road, London NW1 3BH

First published in US 1996 by Contemporary Books, a Division of the McGraw-Hill Companies, 1 Prudential Plaza, 130 East Randolph Street, Chicago, IL 60601, USA.

The 'Teach Yourself' name and logo are registered trade marks of Hodder & Stoughton Ltd.

Typeset by Transet Limited, Coventry, England.
Printed in Great Britain for Hodder & Stoughton Educational, a division of Hodder Headline Ltd., 338 Euston Road, London NW1 3BH by Cox & Wyman Ltd, Reading, Berkshire.

Impression number   7 6 5 4 3 2 1
Year   2009 2008 2007 2006 2005 2004
                               2003

contents

Dedication
For Garry, Chloé and Thomas

introduction

Massage is an instinctive therapy that everyone has the ability to learn. The aim of this book is to encourage your natural abilities and give you the knowledge and expertise to practise safely and effectively on your family and friends. The information contained in these chapters will also be useful to the student or practising therapist, particularly the very comprehensive section on muscles in the appendix.

You employ your innate ability to touch therapeutically in your daily life. If you have a headache, you instinctively rub around the neck and the temples to soothe away the pain and tension. If you hurt your knee or bang your elbow, your first reaction is to massage it to relieve the pain. Children will hold and rub their tummies when they have stomach-ache and eventually the pain will go. A parent feels a child's feverish forehead to check for a high temperature and will massage in response to a child's bumps and cries of pain.

The healing power of therapeutic massage is also used for emotional problems. To comfort distraught friends or relatives you may put your arms around them, hold or stroke them to comfort, support and reassure them in their times of need.

Body and mind should not be regarded as separate entities. Physical symptoms such as headaches or constant fatigue are often an indication of what is 'on our mind'. Muscles contract and tighten in response to anger and anxiety or may become slack as we resign ourselves to what is happening in our lives. Within the physical body is buried a whole lifetime of experience and emotions – birth, childhood, pleasure and pain, shock, frustration, fear, grief, joy and much more besides. Massage is an excellent tool for enabling us to become more aware of what is happening deep within us.

The importance and need for touch is reflected in our everyday language. We talk of being 'deeply touched' when trying to express a reaction. We ask our friends to keep 'in touch' or 'stay in contact' with us. We speak of 'being in touch' or 'out of touch' with our feelings. We describe others as being a 'soft touch' or a bit 'touchy'. We also experience 'gut feelings' about a particular situation.

Touch is essential for our growth and well-being. It is the first sense to be developed in the womb, and early touching while the foetus grows in the womb enhances the development of the nervous system and encourages communication and close bonding between mother and baby. Children need cuddles from their parents to give them a feeling of security and to show them how much they are loved.

01

the history and benefits of massage

In this chapter you will learn:
- about the history of massage
- the benefits of massage.

History

Historical records prove that massage is the oldest form of physical medicine known to humans. The origin of the word 'massage', however, is very unclear. It has been suggested that it may have come from the Arabic word *mash*, which means 'to press softly'. Another theory is that it derives from the Greek word *massein* meaning 'to knead'. It may owe its derivation to the French word *masser* meaning 'to shampoo'.

In China the oldest recorded medical text the *Nei Ching*, written by the Yellow Emperor, includes numerous references to the use of massage for healing purposes. Evidence also comes from Egypt where foot and hand massage is depicted on a wall painting on the physician's tomb in Saqqara dating back to 2330 BC. The traditional Indian system of medicine known as Ayurveda (Ayur = life, veda = knowledge) dating back thousands of years refers to the importance of massage.

There is much evidence that massage was strongly advocated by the Greek and Roman physicians. Socrates, Plato and Heroditus all extolled the virtues of massage. The Greeks and Romans knew about the anatomy and physiology of the human body, and indeed the majority of anatomical terms currently in use are of Greek or Roman origin. In the early fifth century BC the Greek physician Hippocrates, known as the 'father of medicine' wrote that 'rubbing can bind a joint that is too loose and loosen a joint that is too rigid ... hard rubbing binds, much rubbing causes parts to waste and moderate rubbing makes them grow'. The Greek physician Asclepiades combined massage and exercise in his treatments. Pliny, who was a renowned Roman naturalist was regularly massaged to alleviate his asthma. Galen, the Roman Emperor's physician, prescribed massage for the injured gladiators and for preparation for combat in the arenas. Celcus, another Roman physician, advocated massage for pain relief and strengthening limbs. He wrote that 'chronic pains in the head are relieved by rubbing the head itself' and 'a paralyzed limb is strengthened by rubbing'. Julius Caesar, who suffered from neuralgia, was treated daily for this condition and for headaches. After the fall of the Roman Empire little evidence is documented until the Middle Ages. Unfortunately massage suffered at this time as the Church held contempt for the 'pleasures of the body'. Fortunately it re-emerged after the Renaissance. Physicians like the French doctor Ambrose Paré contributed to its re-establishment in the medical world. Massage was considered to be an important part of medicine.

At the beginning of the nineteenth century the Swedish professor, Per Henrik Ling (1776–1839), developed his technique known as 'Swedish Massage'. He established an institute in Stockholm where massage and remedial gymnastics were taught and in 1877 Swedish massage was introduced to the United States by Dr Mitchell. In 1894, in Britain, The Society of Trained Masseuses was established. In 1934 this society changed its title to the Chartered Society of Physiotherapists. Unfortunately with the advent of various electrical treatments, the use of massage gradually began to disappear from the curriculum of the orthodox physiotherapy schools. Massage is less used by physiotherapists in hospitals today. Sadly, hospital physiotherapists simply do not have the time to spend half an hour with each patient – the minimum amount of time required for a massage treatment.

Nowadays massage is becoming increasingly popular and therapists work not only in their private practices and health and beauty clubs, but also in hospitals and hospices. They regard electro-therapy as complementary treatment to their massage work rather than as a supplement. Gradually the rather 'seedy' and sexual image of massage being practised in 'massage parlours' has been transformed. Massage therapists now work alongside the medical professionals and enjoy the respect that they deserve. A well-qualified therapist must undergo a thorough training in anatomy and physiology as well as in massage. Years of experience are then required to develop sensitivity and competency (see taking it further section for training establishments). However, even schools registered with a particular massage body have varied standards and, as usual, 'word-of-mouth' is the best recommendation.

Benefits

Massage is an ancient healing art with enormous benefits for all the systems of the body, some of which are outlined below.

The nervous system is profoundly influenced by the application of massage. The effects of massage may be soothing and sedative, providing relief from nervous irritability. Disorders such as insomnia, tension, headaches and other stress-related conditions respond to the healing power of touch as peace and harmony returns to the troubled mind. Alternatively, the effects of massage on the nerves may be stimulating, promoting an increase in the activity of the muscles, vessels and glands governed by them. It is invaluable in cases of lethargy and fatigue.

The muscular system derives enormous benefits. Muscles maintain a balance in relaxing and contracting. Some massage movements relax and stretch the muscles and soft tissues of the body, reducing muscular tension and cramp. Fibrous tissues, adhesions and old scar tissue can be broken down and cleansed of waste deposits. As muscles contract, toxic products are eliminated. Other movements produce the contraction of muscles promoting good muscle tone. Muscle fatigue and stiffness caused by overactivity, and the resulting build-up of toxic substances in the muscles, is reduced by muscular contraction and relaxation.

The skeletal system is strengthened by using massage. Bone is indirectly affected by massage. Improvements to the circulation of blood and lymph in the muscles lead to better circulation in the underlying bones, benefiting their nutrition and growth. Stiffness of the joints, and pains resulting from conditions such as arthritis, are reduced providing comfort and ease of movement.

The circulatory system also benefits from the action of massage. It takes the pressure off the arteries and veins, accelerating the flow of blood through the system providing relief for poor circulation and cardiac problems. The heartbeat strengthens, the rate of the heartbeat decreases and high blood pressure is reduced.

The lymphatic system is stimulated and the flow of lymph is accelerated throughout the system. As the massage strokes are performed, the waste and poisonous substances which have accumulated in our overstressed bodies are rapidly eliminated. When we sustain injuries, there is often a great deal of oedema (swelling) which should be dispersed into the lymphatic circulation. Massage can empty the lymph vessels and allow the swelling to disperse. If this fluid is not moved on, it becomes semi-solid and thus is unable to pass into lymph vessels. Therefore, it sticks to the surrounding tissues (muscles, bones, tendons, ligaments) and forms what are known as 'adhesions'. If adhesions form in a joint then movement will be restricted permanently.

The respiratory system responds as increased activity in the lungs is stimulated by massage. As the treatment proceeds, the breath slows and deepens. If necessary, mucus and bronchial secretions can be encouraged to leave the lungs by percussive movements on the back and over the lungs.

The digestive system benefits when massage promotes the peristaltic activity (wave-like motion) in the colon enhancing the elimination of faecal matter and combating constipation. It strengthens the muscular walls of the intestines and abdomen, and stimulates the secretion of digestive juices from the liver, pancreas, stomach and intestines. As well as helping the digestion and elimination of food, massage also increases absorption of digested foods.

The skin Both the activity and the nutrition of the skin benefit from massage. The sweat and sebaceous glands are stimulated, improving their function and ensuring the elimination of waste products. As dead skin cells are removed, pores are encouraged to remain open allowing increased skin respiration, suppleness and elasticity. Skin condition, texture and tone are greatly improved – the skin is healthy and glowing following a treatment.

The genito-urinary system The use of abdominal and back massage promotes the activity of the kidneys, which enhances the elimination of waste products and reduces fluid retention.

The reproductive system can also be improved. Abdominal and back massage can help to alleviate menstrual problems such as period pains, irregular menstruation, PMS and the symptoms of menopause.

Massage is an excellent preventive treatment essential for the maintenance of health and fitness. Prevention is always far better than cure. Nowadays people of all ages are increasingly considering natural therapies as a way to encourage an improved sense of well-being and as a means to a long, happy and harmonious life free of illness.

02

setting the scene

In this chapter you will learn:

- how to create the perfect ambience
- which equipment you will need.

It is important to pay attention to the environment where you give your massage treatment. Careful preparation and the right setting will make a good massage even better! Both the giver and receiver should feel relaxed as soon as they arrive. Always ensure that all towels, cushions and oils are on hand so that you will not lose contact and thus break the flow of the massage. A massage should never be hurried.

Peace and quiet

These are vital. Ensure that you choose a time when you will not be disturbed. Intrusions and distractions are extremely disconcerting, breaking your concentration and destroying the flow of your massage movements. Take the telephone off the hook and tell your friends and family not to enter the room. You may decide to choose some soothing background music, although this is a matter of personal preference. Some people will prefer silence. (See 'Useful addresses', p.188, for information on massage/relaxation cassettes.)

Cleanliness

Always wash your hands before as well as after the treatment. Make sure that your fingernails are short and clean – trim them as far down as possible. Do not wear any jewellery on your hands. Rings, bracelets and watches can all scratch the receiver.

Warmth

The room should be draught-free and warm, yet well ventilated. Nothing will destroy a massage more quickly than physical coldness: it is impossible to relax when you feel cold. Heat the room prior to treatment and, as the receiver's body temperature will drop, ensure that you have a good supply of towels. Keep all parts of the receiver's body covered other than the area on which you are working. Warm your hands if they feel cold, either by rubbing them briskly together, or by immersing them in warm water.

Lighting

Soft and subdued lighting will create the ideal atmosphere. Bright lights falling on the receiver's face will not make for a relaxing atmosphere and will cause tension around the eyes. Candlelight provides the perfect setting, or you may wish to use a tinted bulb. Choose from pale pink, blue, green, peach or lavender.

Colour

The most therapeutic colours to have in the room are pastel shades – pale pink, blue, green, lilac or peach decor and towels are perfect for the occasion. Colours such as red will tend to generate anger and restlessness.

Clothes

Wear comfortable and loose-fitting clothes as you need to move around easily and the room in which you will be working will be warm. White is the best colour to wear when giving a massage since it will reflect any negativity (negative emotions) released from the individual being treated. Go barefoot if possible, otherwise wear flat shoes. The receiver should undress down to whatever level is comfortable. Suggest he or she undresses down to at least underwear. Point out that any areas which are not being worked on will be covered up as this will create a sense of security and trust.

Finishing touches

Fresh flowers will scent your room or you could burn some incense or essential oils before the treatment. Refer to Chapter 06 of this book for suggestions. Crystals may also enhance the environment. Rose quartz relaxes and soothes and amethyst is useful for absorbing both physical and emotional negativity. At the end of the treatment a piece of obsidian, haematite, black tourmaline or smoky quartz can be used to 'ground' the receiver.

Equipment

Massage surface

You may work on the floor using a firm yet well-padded surface. This will allow you to give a massage wherever you want. Place a large, thick piece of foam or two or three blankets or a thick duvet on the floor. Use plenty of cushions during the massage. When the receiver is lying on the back (supine position), place one cushion under the head and one under the knees to take the pressure off the lower back (see Figure 2.1).

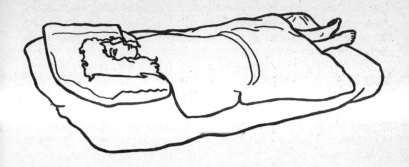

figure 2.1   supine position for working with receiver lying on the back

When the receiver is lying on the front (prone position), place a cushion under the feet, one under the head and shoulders and one under the abdomen if you wish (see Figure 2.2).

Ensure that you have something to kneel on to avoid sore knees. If you are unfortunate enough to suffer from a bad back or have knee problems it may be a good idea to invest in a portable couch. It is far less tiring and you can reach the receiver's body more easily. You could improvise by using the kitchen table, if the height is comfortable for you.

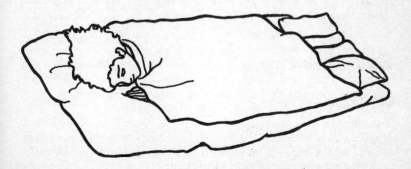

figure 2.2   prone position for working with receiver lying face down

Never use a bed as most are far too soft and wide for massage purposes and any pressure you apply will be absorbed by the mattress.

Carrier oils

I believe that the only really effective way to massage is with oil. Your hands will glide smoothly over the skin and the movements will flow freely. Oils also prevent skin abrasions. Do not leave large amounts of oil on the receiver's skin at the end of the massage. Some people prefer to use talcum powder as a medium, but I find it restrictive, and it is unpleasant for both giver and receiver to inhale the powder.

Some people object to the use of any sort of medium, but massage without any medium can be uncomfortable, and movements are not as smooth, particularly in the case of a hairy individual. In addition, oil massage makes the skin smooth and soft. As opinions vary so much, I advise you to use whatever medium you feel comfortable with.

The carrier oil (also known as base oil or fixed oil) you choose should always be of vegetable origin and also cold pressed (not removed by chemicals), unrefined and additive free. Cold pressed, unrefined carrier oils contain vitamins, minerals and fatty acids and, therefore, nourish the skin. The more highly processed the vegetable oils are, the less vitamin content will be retained. I do not recommend the use of mineral oil, such as commercial baby oil, because it is not as easily absorbed. Vegetable oil molecules are easily absorbed through the skin pores, whereas mineral oil tends to clog the pores.

It is a good idea to mix several different base oils together for a therapeutic formula. The lighter vegetable oils may be used unblended if you wish (e.g. sweet almond, apricot kernel, peach kernel, grapeseed) or they may constitute the highest proportion of the massage blend. The thicker, richer oils, which are usually more expensive, may be added to improve absorption and nourish the skin. The thicker oils tend to be too heavy and sticky when used on their own in a full treatment. This is my favourite recipe for a special carrier oil blend:

To a 100 ml bottle add

one teaspoon (approximately 5 ml) apricot kernel oil
one teaspoon avocado pear oil
one teaspoon calendula oil
one teaspoon evening primrose oil
one teaspoon jojoba oil
one teaspoon peach kernel oil
one teaspoon wheatgerm oil

Fill up the bottle with sweet almond oil

The carrier oils in my 'special blend' are all are highly therapeutic in their own right.

Sweet almond oil (*Prunus amygdalis*)
Contains many vitamins, minerals and fatty acids and is useful for all skin types. It is particularly good for dry, sensitive, inflamed or prematurely aged skin. It can be used on its own as a base oil. Sweet almond oil is popular and is often used as the highest proportion of a massage blend. It is a pale yellow, low-odour oil much favoured by the beauty industry – it was used by Napoleon's wife Josephine!

Apricot kernel (*Prunus armenica*) and peach kernel oil (*Prunus persica*)
Excellent for all skin types. Their nourishing properties make them an ideal choice for a facial oil, particularly where the skin is dry or sensitive. Although I add them to my blend they could be used unblended, although they are more expensive than sweet almond oil as they are produced in smaller quantities.

Avocado pear oil (*Persea americana*)
Has a wonderful dark green colour if it is unrefined and contains vitamin D, lecithin and fatty acids. It penetrates well in spite of its thickness, and is healing and soothing for all skin types. Dry, dehydrated skin, wrinkled skin and eczema particularly will benefit. It normally constitutes 10 per cent or less of a blend.

Calendula oil (*Calendula officinalis*)
Has anti-inflammatory, astringent, hormonal, healing and soothing properties. It is particularly suitable for eczema, psoriasis, rashes, broken and thread veins, varicose veins, wounds, scars, bedsores, bruises and sensitive skin. Calendula cream is popular among homoeopaths. Calendula oil would normally make up 10 per cent of a blend.

Evening primrose oil (*Oenothera biennis*)
Increasingly popular, although it is expensive. It contains a therapeutic ingredient known as gamma linoleic acid (GLA) as well as vitamin and minerals. It is recommended for relieving PMS (pre-menstrual syndrome), menopausal problems, MS (multiple sclerosis), heart disease, high cholesterol levels, eczema and psoriasis. It is excellent for regenerating and stimulating the skin. Normally use up to 10 per cent in a blend. Evening primrose oil is often administered internally in capsule form.

Jojoba oil (*Simmondsia chinensis*)

A thick, yellow oil rich in protein and minerals. It nourishes, moisturizes and penetrates deeply and is wonderful as a face or a hair oil. Acne, eczema, dry skin conditions, inflammatory conditions, psoriasis and indeed all skin types will derive benefit from jojoba oil. As a rule up to a 10 per cent blend is used.

Wheatgerm oil (*Triticum vulgare*)

A rich, orange-brown colour oil, invaluable to any blend. It is anti-oxidant and, therefore, prevents the oil from becoming rancid. An ideal preservative. It contains protein, minerals, vitamins and is particularly renowned for its vitamin E content. Its nourishing properties are useful to combat prematurely ageing skin, eczema and psoriasis. It also helps to prevent stretch marks. It is usually added up to 10 per cent in a blend.

Buying base oils

Carrier oils vary widely in price: evening primrose oil costs far more than sweet almond oil (see 'Useful addresses', p.188, for suppliers of pure, high quality carrier oils).

Always look for 'cold pressed' vegetable carrier oils. The virgin oil is of the highest quality as it comes from the first pressing and has the highest vitamin and mineral content. After the first pressing, the base oil may be treated with heat or synthetically to remove colour or aroma and the vitamin and mineral content will be drastically reduced. The best base oils which are 'cold pressed' will usually have a rich colour and a characteristic aroma.

When blending essential oils with a carrier oil, the essential oil content is usually between 1 per cent and 3 per cent. Approximately 20 drops of essential oil is equivalent to 1 ml. Therefore, a 1 per cent essential oil content would be:

2 drops to 10 mls
10 drops to 50 mls
20 drops to 100 mls

Pure essential oils may be added to the carrier oil in order to enhance the treatment (see Chapter 05 on aromatherapy and also *Teach Yourself Aromatherapy*).

Always keep the oil within easy reach during the treatment. Do not use too much oil as you will be unable to make proper contact and the receiver will feel most uncomfortable and sticky. A complete treatment actually requires only a few teaspoons of oil. Warm the oil before the massage.

Never pour oil directly on to the body. Pour about 2 ml (half a teaspoon) on to the palm of one hand and then rub your hands together to warm the oil slightly before applying it. When you require more lubricant keep one hand in contact with the body. Breaking contact destroys the continuity of the massage and creates a feeling of insecurity.

Contraindications (when not to massage)

High temperature/fevers
The body is already fighting off toxins as indicated by the rise in temperature. A massage would release even more unwelcome toxins into the system.

Infectious and contagious diseases
These include ringworm, scabies, impetigo and chicken pox – you do not want to spread the condition or transfer it to yourself. Conditions such as acne, psoriasis and eczema are not infectious and may improve with the use of essential oils such as lavender (refer to *Teach Yourself Aromatherapy* in this series for information on specific skin conditions). Massage is also contraindicated over an area of sepsis such as a boil or carbuncle.

Thrombo-phlebitis and other similar conditions
Phlebitis is inflammation of a vein. The skin near the inflamed vein is red, hot and swollen. The patient experiences considerable pain and tenderness to the touch along the vein. If a clot (thrombus) forms in the vein, massage is contraindicated since the clot could move, resulting in death.

Advanced varicose veins
You risk the danger here of causing further inflammation and great pain.

Recent scars or operations
Beware of recent scars and open wounds. Old scar tissue **can** be massaged.

Abdomen during pregnancy
Although massage is extremely beneficial during pregnancy only light massage should be applied to the abdominal area and lower back. Where there is a history of risk of miscarriage take particular care during the first three months.

Lumps and unexplained pain

These may be innocent but it is wise to have them investigated by a doctor. Indeed any condition that creates doubt in your mind should be investigated by a doctor to exclude the possibility of serious disease. If in doubt – check it out!

Inflammatory conditions e.g. bursitis (housemaid's knee)

Signs of inflammation include redness, heat, swelling, tenderness, pain and loss of movement. Inflamed organs should also never be massaged (e.g. gastro-enteritis).

Drugs

After a cortisone injection do not massage heavily over the site of the injection as pressure on muscles with cortisone in them can make the fibres fall apart. Allow approximately six or eight weeks to elapse.

Patients on certain medications such as steroids and blood thinning drugs may have thin skin and bruise easily. Only light massage should be used on such individuals.

Cancer and massage

There is a great deal of confusion and fear surrounding massage and cancer, and there are still many questions that need to be answered. It is interesting that some oncology (cancer) units in hospitals now have massage therapists. It is no longer the case that massage is only offered in hospices at the final stages of cancer. In cancer patients gentle massage will have many benefits. Aches and pains may be considerably relieved as the body produces endorphines (pain relievers) in response to the stimulus of touch. Stress, tension and insomnia may be relieved and after a good night's sleep it is much easier to cope and put things in perspective. Anticipatory nausea evoked by the fear and dread prior to chemotherapy can be helped by massage given before the treatment.

Massage encourages a positive body image – a woman who has had a mastectomy may feel unfeminine and disfigured; massage will allow her to feel a whole person once again.

Constipation, a common side effect of the opiate group of painkillers, such as codeine, can also be alleviated by the use of abdominal massage (**unless there is active disease in this area**).

You should never massage over the site of a tumour. Avoid current radiotherapy sites for two weeks after the last treatment. All the usual contraindications I have already outlined should also, of course, be taken into account.

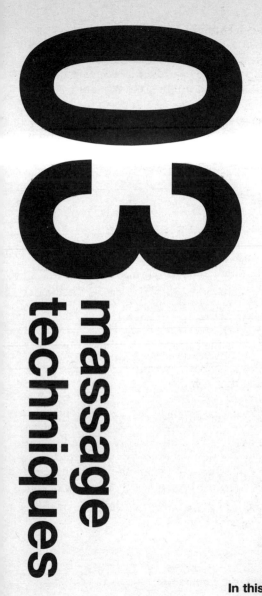

03

massage techniques

In this chapter you will learn:
- how to master the basic massage techniques
- the benefits of each movement
- common errors to avoid
- hand exercises to improve flexibility, strength and heighten sensitivity.

Massage can be simple! Even though there is a wide variety of different massage movements, most techniques are merely a variation on the strokes explained below. With the aid of these basic movements, you will be able to perform a complete body massage. As you develop and gain confidence, you will invent your own strokes to build up an extensive repertoire. Please read the contraindications carefully in Chapter 02 before you begin. Some of the illustrations have the symbol ➲ to show the position of the receiver's head.

Effleurage/Stroking

Description

Effleurage (stroking) is one of the principal movements of massage and may be performed on any area of the body. It signals the beginning and the end of a massage both preceding and succeeding all other strokes and facilitating the flow from one movement to the next. Initially, it enables the giver to distribute the oil evenly on to the receiver's body. Use the palms of both hands as you glide over the surface of the skin moulding your hands to the contours of the body. You should keep as much of the hands as possible in contact with the body. The receiver experiences one continuous movement as you apply firm rhythmic pressure on the upward stroke yet glide downwards to your starting point with a featherlight touch (see Figure 3.1). Maintain an even rhythm and avoid jerky movements at all times. Pressure can be superficial or deep according to the effect required. Close your eyes as you effleurage to accentuate and heighten your sensitivity and sense of touch. Experiment with different depths of pressure. Where the area to be treated is small (e.g. the face) use the pads of the palmar surface of your fingers or thumbs.

Benefits

- The receiver experiences an immediate sense of well-being and relaxation.
- A relationship of trust is established between the two of you as your hands become accustomed to the receiver's body.
- Stroking enables you to familiarize yourself with the amount of pressure to apply.
- Effleurage provides a link between techniques.

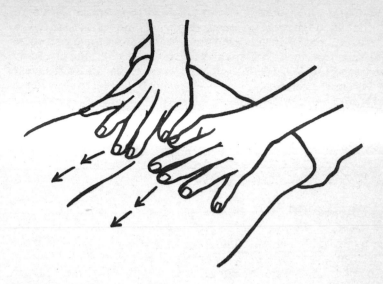

figure 3.1 effleurage of the back

- Effleurage, when performed slowly, has a sedative action and is particularly beneficial for soothing the nerves. Stress and strain may be relieved, tension headaches dispelled and patterns of insomnia broken.
- Use brisk effleurage to enliven, revive and stimulate the central nervous system.
- The tissues will warm up as you stroke the body, improving the circulation.
- The flow of lymph is increased, helping to get rid of waste and poisonous substances.
- Effleurage improves the skin, encouraging a healthy and glowing complexion.

Errors to avoid

- Do not lose contact with the receiver (loss of contact means loss of confidence and loss of relaxation).
- Relax your hands and flow, avoiding any jerky or sudden movements (jerky movements cause jangled nerves). The movements must be rhythmic, smooth and even.
- Use your whole hand and not just the fingertips (you can cover a much wider area), except when working on small areas.

- **No** pressure whatsoever on the downward stroke (effleurage is always performed towards the heart – up the legs, and arms, and up the back). It can also be applied in a centripetal direction (in a circle travelling towards the centre) or in a centrifugal direction (in a circle travelling outwards away from the centre).

Remember
If in doubt, effleurage! Everyone adores this stroke

Friction

Description

Friction movements normally make use of the balls of the thumbs (although the fingertips, knuckles or even the elbows may be used). The muscle is moved against the bone by small circular movements of the balls of the thumbs. Stand directly over the area to be treated and use your body weight to penetrate right down into the deeper tissues – the human body is not as delicate and fragile as you might imagine. This stroke is particularly effective when performed on either side of the spine (see Figure 3.2). If your thumbs are not aching by the time you reach the neck area you are not performing the stroke correctly!

Benefits

- This technique is particularly useful for breaking down the knots and nodules that build up in the body due to the stresses and strains of daily life.
- Any accumulated waste products may be eliminated.
- Friction helps to break down the fatty deposits and is therefore of benefit in cases of obesity.
- Friction is very effective around a **well-healed** scar to break down adhesions and is also used to massage around bony prominences such as the patella (knee cap).
- It also increases the temperature by increasing cellular activity and bringing an increased flow of blood to an area providing temporary analgesia (pain relief).

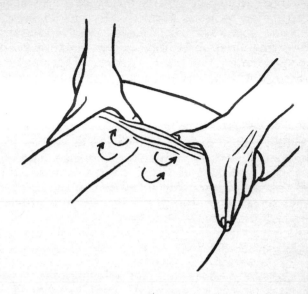

figure 3.2 friction of the back working from the base of the spine towards the neck

Errors to avoid

- Work deeper and deeper into the tissues **gradually**, as the pain tolerance levels vary greatly. Do not overtreat an area as this can lead to pain and soreness.
- Do not hunch your shoulders with the effort (otherwise **you** will need a massage yourself straight afterwards).
- Ensure that you are moving the tissues **under** the skin and not **just** the skin.
- Use the pads of the thumbs only, avoiding digging the nails in!

Petrissage

Description

This stroke referred to as petrissage (derived from 'pétrir' meaning 'to knead'). Petrissage can be subdivided into picking-up, wringing, squeezing and rolling. If you are good at kneading dough then you will quickly become an expert!

It is an extremely powerful and vigorous movement, which enables you to work deeply on the muscles. You may apply it to every area of the body, except for the face, and it is effective on the fleshy areas such as the hips and thighs. In **picking-up**, place your hands flat on the part being treated and grasp the muscle (not the skin) firmly with one or both hands, then pull it as far away as possible from the bone.

Once you have picked up the muscle you may **squeeze** it gently. Squeezing is particularly effective in alleviating muscle spasm. You may now **roll** the muscle in both directions – your thumbs may roll the muscle towards your fingers or your fingers may roll the muscle towards your thumbs. **Wringing** is a variation on picking-up. It is picking-up with a twist! The muscle is picked up and then pulled towards you and 'wrung' out. Imagine that you are wringing out a towel or a chamois leather (see Figure 3.3, showing the technique on a thigh).

Benefits

- By alternately squeezing and relaxing, the veins and lymphatic vessels are emptied and filled, bringing fresh nutrients to the muscles.
- Any toxins that have accumulated are removed from the deeper tissues.

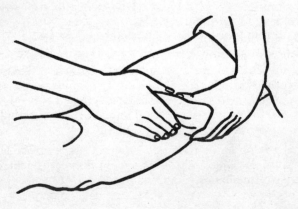

figure 3.3   wringing the back of the thigh

- Petrissage is invaluable in helping to break down and remove fatty deposits around the thighs, shoulders and buttocks.
- It also helps to prevent muscle stiffness after exercise and can relieve muscle spasm.

Errors to avoid

- Make sure that you use the whole of your hand rather than just your fingers and your thumbs;
- Pick up the muscle and **not** the skin otherwise there is the danger of pinching the flesh. Do not slide your fingers over the receiver's skin.

Percussion movements/tapotement

Description

Percussion movements (tapotement) involve a series of light, brisk, striking actions applied with alternate hands in rapid succession. Two of the main percussion strokes are **cupping** and **hacking**; they may be performed on many areas of the body, although they are especially effective when used on fleshy and large muscular areas of the body such as the thighs. Other tapotement movements include **flicking, beating** and **pounding.** When performing tapotement movements the action originates from the wrists and not from the elbows or shoulders, which remain still throughout. Many beginners make the mistake of practising percussion movements from the elbows and shoulders, resulting in frustration and clumsiness.

Cupping is performed with your palms facing downwards, forming a hollow curve. It is sometimes known as 'clapping' (see Figure 3.4). As you bring your cupped hands down on to the body in quick succession, a vacuum is created which is released when you bring your hands up. The sound should be hollow like a horse trotting. Listen for the sound.

Hacking is probably the best-known massage stroke since it is the movement almost always shown in films. It is achieved with the edge of the hands (the ulnar border). Hold your hands over the body with the palms facing each other, the thumbs uppermost (see Figure 3.5). Flick your hands rhythmically up and down in rapid succession. Use these movements at the end of a massage to wake the person up! Obviously, if you are trying

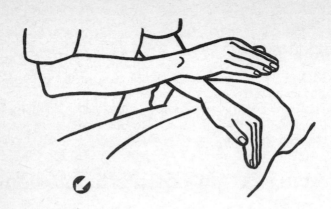

figure 3.4 cupping the sides of the back

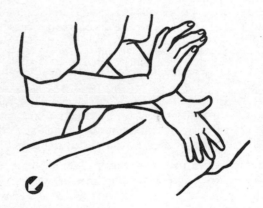

figure 3.5 hacking the sides of the back

to relax someone totally hacking may be omitted altogether. If you are nervous about using these movements, practise them first on a cushion or a pillow placed on your lap.

Flicking is a movement similar to hacking and is often described as 'finger hacking'. To perform this movement flex your wrists slightly and bring only the sides of your little fingers into contact with the body (not the edge of the hands as well). Flicking is a much lighter, softer movement than the usual hacking movement.

Beating and pounding movements are both applied with your hands in a closed position with your fists **lightly** clenched. Beating is performed with the ulnar border (little finger side) of the closed fists, whereas in pounding the palmar surface of the hands are employed. The closed fists are applied to the body in quick succession.

Benefits

- Percussion movements are very stimulating. Tapotement is extremely useful for athletes before an event.
- As the blood is drawn to the surface the circulation is improved.
- Cupping is beneficial when performed over the upper and middle back area as it loosens mucus in the lungs aiding expectoration.
- Percussion movements are also valuable in inducing muscle tone as well as strengthening muscles since they stimulate the muscle to contract.
- They are also useful in reducing fatty deposits and flabby muscle areas and are often used over the buttocks and thighs.
- Gentle tapotement given over the abdomen increases peristalsis, thereby aiding conditions such as constipation.

Errors to avoid

- Make sure that when cupping, your hands are really cupped – otherwise a smacking sound will be heard, which is stinging and painful.
- When hacking do not tense up the fingers of your hands or the movement will feel like a karate chop.
- Keep your hands relaxed and loose and ensure that the movements are coming **from the wrist**. Keep your elbows tucked closely in; if you use your elbows and shoulders you will be exhausted quickly.
- These strokes must **not** be performed over the bony areas – they will hurt.
- Try not to concentrate on the strokes, otherwise you may lose the rhythm.

Vibration and shaking

Description

Vibration is a fine, gentle trembling movement of the tissues, which is performed by your hand or fingers. **Shaking** is a larger movement performed more vigorously.

To perform vibration place the palmar surface of your hand on the part of the body or the limb to be treated. Vibrate the entire muscle area rapidly. The movement may either be gentle, in which case it is known as 'vibration', or vigorous, which is referred to as 'shaking'. Gentle vibration can be performed using just the fingertips along the course of a nerve.

Benefits

- Vibration along the course of a nerve is helpful for restoring and maintaining the functions of a nerve and the muscles supplied by them, thereby improving their nutrition. It is particularly useful in cases of paralysis or where there is loss of nerve power.
- Vibrating and shaking can be performed on the abdominal area to aid digestion and relieve flatulence. It can be used to promote tone in the colon and to combat constipation.
- Vibration and shaking over the thoracic area and chest is particularly beneficial for respiratory problems such as asthma, sometimes in combination with the tapotement movements.

Errors to avoid

- Do not perform vibration and shaking where there is inflammation.
- Do not apply too much pressure.

Exercises for your hands

It is essential to exercise your hands in order to improve flexibility, increase strength, heighten sensitivity and achieve an expert touch.

To increase flexibility and strength

1 Hold a small rubber ball in your hand and squeeze and relax your fingers around the ball repeatedly. Now exercise the other hand in the same way.

2 Gently pull and stretch out the thumb and fingers of each hand one by one. Then circle each one carefully.

3 Place your hands face down and shake them out from the wrists as loosely and as rapidly as possible.

4 With fingers relaxed, circle both wrists clockwise and anticlockwise. You can also perform this movement with your fists clenched.

5 With hands relaxed, bend each joint and slowly close each hand into a fist with the thumb outside the fingers. You can also perform this movement rapidly ensuring that a fist is made each time.

6 Throw out your fingers so that they are separated and extended as far as possible. Repeat at least ten times.

7 Tuck your elbows closely into your waist and rotate your loose wrists and forearms quickly in both directions.

8 Place the palms of your hands together in a prayer position. Rapidly rub your hands together in a backwards and forwards motion. Notice the heat produced by this movement.

9 Practise hacking and cupping on a cushion, remembering to keep your elbows closely tucked in and gradually building up speed.

To increase sensitivity

1 Bring the palms of your hands close to each other so that they are almost touching. Close your eyes and take note of unusual sensations such as tingling, heat, vibrations or pulsation. Now slowly separate your hands until they are about 5 cm (2 inches) apart. Then return them to the original position and again note any sensations. Now expand the gap to about 10 cm (4 inches) and then to 15 cm (6 inches), all the time observing any reactions.

2 Ask a partner to sit opposite you. Place your hands approximately 5 cm (3 inches) away from his or her body, starting at the head. Move your hands slowly and steadily down the body to scan the energy field. You may feel temperature changes, tingling, vibrations, pulsations or electric shock type sensations. Repeat this exercise with your

hands about 20 cm (8 inches) away from the person to be scanned.

3 Place a coin under a magazine and with your eyes closed try to find the coin by careful palpation of the upper surface of the magazine. If this is too difficult at first, place the coin under a few sheets of paper and then try to sense its position. Gradually increase the thickness of the barrier between your fingers and the coin until you can find the coin under a telephone directory!

4 Place a human hair under a piece of paper and with your eyes closed try to sense it under the page. Once you can do this easily, place the hair under several pages and repeat the exercise.

5 Place a selection of objects made of different materials (e.g. clay, rubber, plastic, metal, wood) in front of you. With your eyes closed pick up each one in turn and feel the different shapes, texture and flexibility of each item.

6 Sit opposite a partner at a table. Ask your partner to rest one or both arms in a relaxed position on the table. Place one of your hands on to your partner's forearm and the other hand on the table. Focus your attention on what you are feeling. Sense the contrast between living tissue and non-living. You may even feel your hand being 'drawn' towards a certain area of the forearm, wrist or upper arm – if there has been an injury at some time this will still manifest in the tissues.

When performing these exercises ensure that you concentrate fully and use light and slow pressure to get maximum sensory input. Relax your hands as much as possible – rigid, hard hands are not nearly as effective.

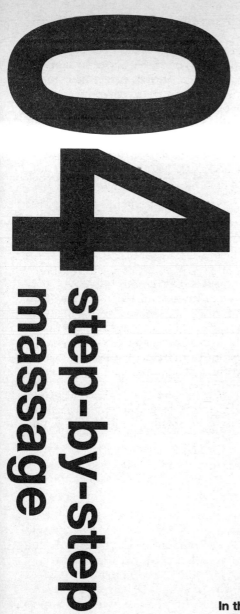

04

step-by-step massage

In this chapter you will learn:
• how to perform a complete
  full body massage: back of
  the leg – back, neck and
  shoulders – foot – front of the
  leg – abdomen – arm and
  hand – chest and neck – face.

Now that you have mastered the basic techniques, this chapter will enable you to carry out a complete full body massage on your family and friends. The complete sequence should take you up to an hour and a half, and it will take you step by step through the whole body. However, if time is limited, it is far more therapeutic to concentrate on just a few areas, rather than trying to rush your way through an entire massage. It is quite possible to spend an hour on the back alone. As you become familiar with the various movements I urge you to work intuitively discovering and experimenting with new techniques to develop your own style.

If you are intending to use massage professionally, formal training with a reputable establishment is vital (see 'Useful addresses', p.188). A thorough grounding in anatomy and physiology will be given in addition to the practical tuition. Before embarking on any course always check that it is recognised by a professional body and leads to a diploma, and that it has adequate insurance cover.

If you would like to study massage it is essential to learn basic anatomy, the names of the main muscles of the body and their functions. In the 'Taking it further' section you will find useful terminology for describing the actions of muscles and basic anatomy of all the main body areas. Also included is extensive and detailed information of all the major muscles of the body together with fully labelled diagrams. This material provides a comprehensive vital reference guide for the student and professional massage therapist. I have tried to keep the language as simple as possible, making it as accessible and appealing to the interested lay-person as to the student of massage or sports therapy.

Before you begin ensure that you have created the right environment (see Chapter 02) and that you have everything you need within easy reach. Always check carefully for any contraindications (see pages 15–16).

Always be aware of your posture. Whether you are working on the floor or at a table, keep your back relaxed yet straight throughout the massage. When standing bend your knees and tuck your bottom in so that your back can work from a secure base (i.e. the pelvis). Allow your thighs to do most of the work – not your back. Remember that it should be as relaxing to give a massage as it is to receive one. With practice you will learn to avoid tensing your muscles so that the healing energy can flow freely through your hands and body. If you do not pay attention to your posture you will quickly become tired. Habits are difficult to break so if you consciously control your posture now instead of slumping it will become automatic later on. Your shoulders, arms and lower back will thus take as little strain as possible. If you are using a couch, stand close to it so that you need only do a minimum amount of reaching.

Ensure that your state of mind is calm when giving a massage. The quality and success of a treatment depends upon this. Do not attempt to give a massage when you are feeling angry, moody, depressed or unwell. Your negativity will be transmitted. Your attention must be devoted entirely to the receiver. If you are worrying about your own problems and your mind is drifting, this will be communicated immediately. Ensure that you are aware of your patient's breathing and that you are sensitive to the receiver's reactions. Observe the facial expressions and be aware of any tensing up in the muscles.

Spend time consciously relaxing yourself before the treatment and, most importantly, be guided by your intuition. Take a few deep breaths before the massage allowing all tension and anxiety to flow out of your body. Breathe in peace and breathe out love. Tune in to the person you are massaging. It may help to work with your eyes closed. Give yourself unselfishly to the massage.

If you are very sensitive and intuitive you may find it helpful to 'ground' yourself prior to a treatment. To 'protect' yourself from any negativity, imagine that white, healing light is pouring down from the sky and protecting you as you work.

You are now ready to begin. Good luck!

Back of the body

Back of the leg (posterior leg massage)

The benefits of leg massage
Leg massage is of great benefit, particularly after standing all day at work or after wearing high heels. Leg massage will improve the circulation and help to prevent varicose veins. It is also excellent for the lymphatic system. There may be swelling at the back of the knee (where there are lymph nodes) and also at the ankles. We always massage **up** the legs towards the lymph glands in the groin area to reduce this fluid. Treatment of the back of the legs often helps to alleviate problems in the lower back. Tightness in the upper thigh muscles is usually linked with low back pain. Leg massage is also useful both as a prelude to exercise and afterwards to prevent stiffness.

But do not:

- use **heavy** pressure over varicose veins or where a person has thin skin and/or bruises easily (e.g. diabetics and the elderly)
- use **heavy** pressure on the delicate area at the back of the knee (the popliteal space)
- work on inflamed or swollen areas
- work over **recent** scar tissue
- work over infectious skin conditions
- massage where there is thrombo-phlebitis.

The massage
Position yourself at the receiver's feet

1 *Effleuraging the leg*
Effleurage the entire leg moulding your hands to the leg. Apply most of the pressure with the palms of your hands and hardly any pressure to the back of the knee (see Figure 4.1). Hold your hands in a V-shape with one hand in front of the other or cup your hands to perform the stroking movement. Apply pressure only on the upward movements. As your hands reach the top of the thigh separate them and let them glide gently down the sides of the leg to the ankle with **no** pressure. Gradually increase your upward pressure, checking that the patient is comfortable. Perform this effleurage **gently** and **slowly** on individuals who are nervous or who need relaxation. Perform brisk effleurage where stimulation is required (e.g. prior to a sporting activity).

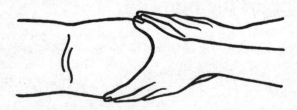

figure 4.1   effleurage the whole leg

2 *Effleuraging the calf*
Effleurage the calf muscles only, evenly and rhythmically, but avoid the popliteal space at the back of the knee.

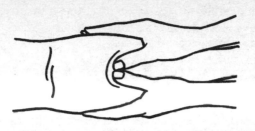

figure 4.2 divide the gastrocnemius muscle of the calf

3 *Splitting the gastrocnemius (belly-shaped muscle)*

Starting at the heel use both thumbs to divide the two heads of the gastrocnemius muscle in the calf (refer to the 'Taking it further' section). Release your pressure just below the back of the knee and glide your hands gently back down to the ankle with no pressure. Repeat this movement several times and feel the muscle fibres separating under your fingers (see Figure 4.2).

4 *Kneading movements*

Position yourself at the side of the receiver's calf to perform the kneading movements. These movements will release any toxins that have accumulated in the deeper tissues and the increased blood supply to the area will carry fresh nutrients to the muscles. Regular effleurage and kneading of the leg muscles is also effective in preventing cramp.

Kneading 1 – pick up and squeeze

Place both hands **flat** on the calf muscles and pick up, squeeze and release the muscles gently (see Figure 4.3). Ensure that you are using the whole of your hands. The receiver will feel an unpleasant 'pinching' sensation if you use only your fingers and thumbs.

Kneading 2 – pick up and roll

Squeeze and pick up the calf muscles again and then roll the muscles in both directions. Using your thumbs, roll the muscle towards your fingers and then, using your fingers, roll the muscle towards your thumbs (see Figure 4.4).

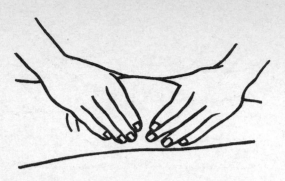

figure 4.3 pick up and squeeze the calf muscles

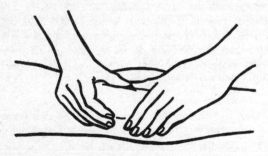

figure 4.4 roll the calf muscles with your thumbs towards your fingers

Kneading 3 – wringing

Place both hands flat on the calf. With alternate hands moving in opposite directions, pick up, squeeze and roll the muscles (see Figure 4.5).

5 Completion of lower leg

Effleurage away any toxins that have been released towards the lymph glands in the groin (the inguinal lymph glands).

6 Effleuraging the thigh

Effleurage the whole of the thigh using firm pressure on the way up and no pressure on the return stroke.

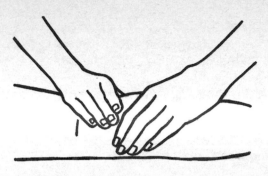

figure 4.5   wring the muscles of the calf

7 *Kneading the thigh*

Pick up, roll and wring the inner, middle and outer thigh muscles (see Figure 4.6). Regular massage of the thigh muscles is invaluable for breaking down the fatty deposits that accumulate around the thighs, and can help to remove cellulite if combined with a sensible diet.

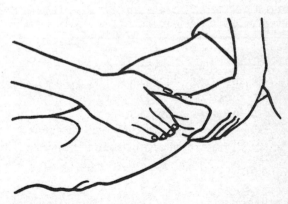

figure 4.6   wring the thigh

8 *Percussion movements*

Perform cupping and hacking over the whole leg, apart from the popliteal space (back of the knee). These movements will stimulate the circulation and encourage muscle tone. For an even stronger effect you can beat and pound the thighs to help to reduce fatty deposits.

9 Completion

To complete the back of the leg, effleurage the entire leg, gliding your hands back with no pressure. Gradually decrease the pressure with each movement. Rest your cupped hands around the heel to signal that you have finished the posterior leg massage.

Repeat on the other leg

Back

The benefits of back massage

Everyone will derive enormous benefits from back massage, irrespective of age. You will be amazed at the number of 'knots' that are discovered during a back treatment. Poor posture, physical or emotional stress, maintaining an unaccustomed position for too long (e.g. gardening), too much sport, excessive studying or a sedentary lifestyle are just some of the factors that can give rise to problems.

Most people will experience a back problem at some time in their life and many back conditions are responsive to massage. However, if the back pain is severe and persistent then always consult a doctor or a fully qualified osteopath. (See 'Useful addresses', p.188). Realignment of the vertebrae may be necessary.

But do not:

- work on infectious skin conditions
- massage directly over **recent** scar tissue
- work on inflamed or swollen areas
- use friction movements directly over the spine
- use heavy pressure where the skin is thin or bruises easily
- massage over lumps and bumps – check these with a doctor first.

The massage

The receiver should lie in a prone position with one pillow beneath the feet to prevent friction of the toes on the couch, one pillow beneath the head and shoulders and a third pillow under the abdomen if necessary. The receiver will find this position comfortable as it allows all the muscles of the body to relax fully.

If the receiver is pregnant or suffers from a condition that makes lying in the prone position impossible then a side-lying position may be adopted (see Chapter 06).

The receiver's arms should be at his or her sides or may hang over the edge of the massage couch. The head may be turned to one side but, if this is painful, place the forehead on the hands. The lower half of the body should be covered with a towel and the towel should be tucked into the underwear.

1 Effleuraging the entire back

Position yourself beside the receiver and begin to effleurage. Start with both hands in the lower back/buttock area, one hand on either side of the spine, fingers pointing towards the head and effleurage upwards towards the neck. As your hands reach the top of the back spread them outwards across the shoulders (see Figure 4.7). To complete the effleurage movement return to the original position, letting your hands glide back without any pressure. Repeat this movement several times to induce relaxation, to establish your own rhythm and to accustom the receiver to your hands. Close your eyes to heighten sensitivity. Gradually increase your pressure with each movement.

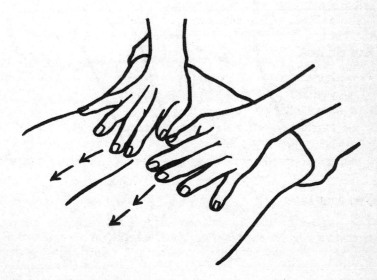

figure 4.7 effleurage the back

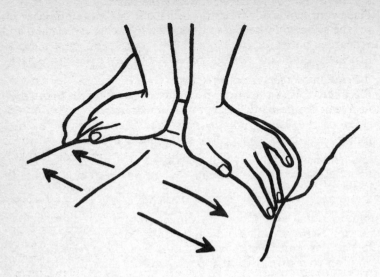

figure 4.8 effleurage outwards across the back

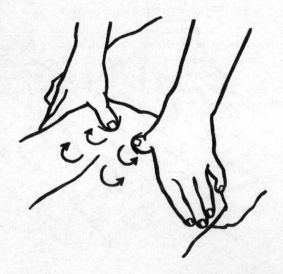

figure 4.9 friction up the back from the base of the spine to the neck

2 *Lateralizing effleurage to the whole back*

Place your hands down flat on either side of (but not directly on to) the spine with the heels of your hands facing each other, and effleurage outwards (see Figure 4.8). Repeat this movement as necessary, gradually working upwards to cover the entire back.

3 *Friction to the spinal muscles*

Place the balls of your thumbs in the two dimples that should be visible at the base of the spine and simultaneously friction both sides of the spinal muscles. Do not perform these friction movements directly on to the spine itself. Proceed up towards the top of the shoulders maintaining the same distance between the thumbs as you travel up the back (see Figure 4.9). Your outward circles should be slow, firm, deep and penetrating as you search out the knots and nodules. If you are performing these movements correctly your thumbs will undoubtedly ache by the time you reach the neck area. Allow your hands to return to the starting point with a featherlight touch. You can friction the spinal muscles several times. Where knots are present perform friction circles over them to try to break them down.

4 *Spinal thumb gliding*

Place the balls of your thumbs in the dimples again and glide your thumbs up towards the neck with firm pressure. Keep your hands in light contact on the return stroke. You can repeat this movement several times to eliminate toxins.

5 *Ironing the spinal muscles*

Starting from the buttocks area work up one side of the back using pushing ironing movements with alternate hands. Follow the movements through with your forearms, working up and over the shoulders and back down again (see Figure 4.10). Do not work directly over the spine.

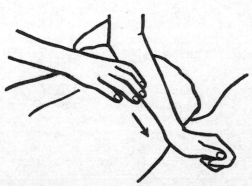

figure 4.10   drain the sides of the back with your hands, wrists and forearms

Repeat these ironing movements on the other side of the back. Do not lose contact as you change your position.

6 *Lateralizing effleurage to the lower back and gluteals (buttocks)*
Repeat step 2 but work only on the lumbar area and buttocks.

7 *Frictioning the iliac crest*
Locate the dimples again and with your thumbs use deep circular friction movements (see Figure 4.11) across the iliac crest (top of the pelvis).

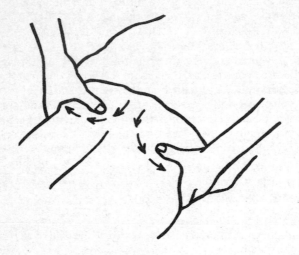

figure 4.11   friction around the iliac crest

8 *Circling the gluteals (buttocks)*
Place one of your hands flat on the sacrum, and rest the other hand on top of this hand. Using the whole of your hand, circle around the right buttock and back to the sacrum and then over the left buttock returning to the sacrum. Repeat this movement several times.

9 *Petrissaging the lumbar area and gluteals*
Working from the opposite side of the receiver knead the gluteals and the lower back area. Work into the muscles slowly and thoroughly as you squeeze, roll and wring the buttocks.

Repeat step 9 on the other side

10 *Tapotement*

Cup and hack the buttock area. You can also beat and pound this region with loosely clenched fists, taking care not to strike any area that is not adequately covered with flesh. These movements will help to break down fatty deposits.

11 *Effleurage*

Effleurage the entire back remembering to use firm pressure on the upward stroke, yet flowing back with a featherlight touch.

12 *Shoulder circling*

Place one hand flat on top of the other and using your whole hand make large circular movements on and around the shoulder blade to warm and loosen the area. Stiffness in the shoulder area is always present and may be caused by emotional stress or by occupational stress (e.g. spending long hours sitting at a desk).

13 *Friction to the scapulae*

The receiver should bend and place the arm behind the back, which will make it easier for you to see the shoulder blade. If this is uncomfortable then the arm may be left at the side. Apply deep circular friction movements all round the shoulder blade (see Figure 4.12). As you encounter the knots and nodules try to remove them with a few friction circles. Always ensure that you are not causing too much discomfort.

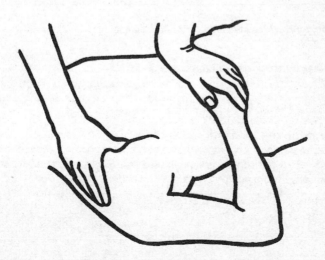

figure 4.12 apply deep friction all around the shoulder blade

Repeat steps 12 and 13 on the other shoulder blade

14 *Petrissaging the shoulders*
Work across the top of the shoulders, rhythmically picking up, squeezing and wringing the trapezius and neighbouring muscles with alternate hands (see Figure 4.13).

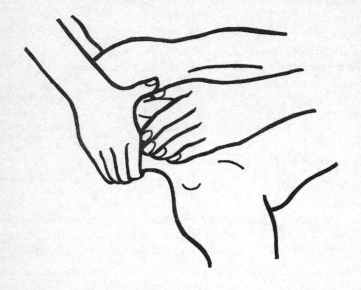

figure 4.13   wring across the top of the shoulders

15 *Draining the shoulder region*
To drain any toxins released into the axilla (armpit) effleurage firmly out and down the inside of the scapulae to the axillary lymph nodes in the armpits.

16 *Loosening the neck*
Ask the receiver to place his or her forehead on to the hands in order to straighten the neck. Roll up a small towel and place it under the forehead for extra comfort. Place both your hands flat down, moulding your hands to the contours of the neck. Pick up and squeeze the neck muscles **slowly** and **gently**. Ensure that you use the whole of your hands and not just the fingers, which will cause an uncomfortable pinching sensation. The neck is a delicate area requiring great care. It is an important area to massage, however, since tension and stiffness in the neck often gives rise to headaches, migraines and even dizziness.

17 *Effleurage*
Effleurage the entire back.

18 *Feathering the back*
Relax your hands and gently stroke them towards you either side of the spine using just your fingertips. Repeat this light downwards stroking movement several times.

19 *Completion*
Completely cover the whole of the back with towels and very gently let your hands come down to rest intuitively on the back. Hold your hands lightly on an area that you feel drawn to.

Ask the receiver to turn over. Place a pillow/cushion under the head and one under the knees to take the pressure off the lower back.

Front of the body

Foot

The benefits of foot massage
Our feet have to support the weight of our entire body and they also act as shock absorbers – no wonder they feel so tired at the end of a hard day! Massage of the feet is marvellous for relaxation and it is remarkable how refreshed and revitalized the whole body feels after a foot massage. Treatment of the feet helps to relieve aches and pains and maintains flexibility and suppleness. Regular foot massage improves the circulation dramatically (feet are often cold) and prevents cramp in the sole of the foot by making sure that the muscles are cleansed of toxins.

But do not:
- use **heavy** pressure on varicose veins or where a person has thin skin and/or bruises easily (e.g. a diabetic)
- massage over **recent** scar tissue or painful areas
- massage directly over contagious skin conditions – for example athlete's foot, verrucae (Chapter 08 covers treatment for these conditions)
- massage firmly on to corns or blisters if it causes pain
- use too much oil as this will make some of the movements impossible to perform.

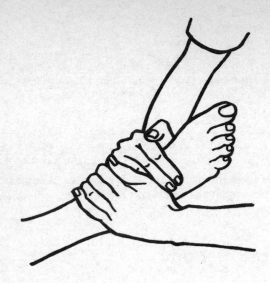

figure 4.14 effleurage the foot

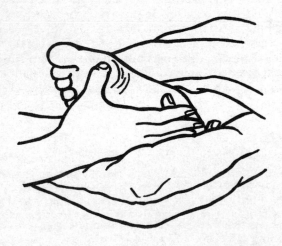

figure 4.15 friction the sole of the foot

The massage

1 *Effleuraging the foot*
Effleurage the whole foot firmly using both hands. Cover the dorsum (top) of the foot, the sides of the foot and the plantar aspect (sole) of the foot. Work from the ends of the toes to the top of the foot (see Figure 4.14). Slide around the ankle bones and glide back.

2 *Frictioning the sole of the foot*
With one hand supporting the heel, friction the entire sole of the foot (see Figure 4.15). Begin underneath the big toe and work outwards towards the little toe. Continue to friction the remainder of the plantar aspect (sole) of the foot in horizontal strips until you have covered the whole area.

3 *Effleurage*
Effleurage the foot.

4 *Frictioning the toes*
Friction the toe joints both top and bottom to loosen them.

5 *Toes*
Supporting the heel with one hand, stretch and circumduct each toe individually.

6 *Effleurage*
Effleurage the foot.

7 *Ankle*
Friction around the ankle joint using both thumbs.

8 *Ankle movements*
Supporting the foot with one hand, slowly but firmly dorsiflex the foot (push it backwards) and plantar flex the foot (point it). Now invert (turn the sole inwards) and evert (turn the sole outwards) the foot. Then circumduct the foot clockwise and anticlockwise.

9 *Vibrations*
Place the palms of your hands one on each side of the foot, and move them alternately and rapidly side to side so that the foot vibrates (see Figure 4.16).

10 *Completion*
Effleurage the foot gently, and to complete the foot massage clasp the foot between both of your hands and squeeze gently.

Repeat on the other foot

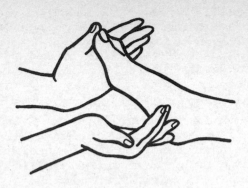

figure 4.16 move the foot rapidly from side to side

Front of the leg (anterior leg massage)

1 *Effleuraging the leg*
Effleurage the entire leg from the ankle to the top of the thigh using only light pressure over the knee. Mould your hands to the contours of the leg. Cup your hands over the front of the ankle, one hand above the other and, as you reach the top of the thigh, separate your hands and glide them gently down the sides of the leg.

2 *Effleuraging the thigh*
Firmly effleurage the whole of the thigh – pressure on the way up, featherlight touch on the return. You are working on the powerful quadriceps muscles and the sartorius on the front of the thigh, the adductors and gracilis on the inner thigh and the tensor fascia lata on the outer aspect of the thigh.

3 *Kneading the thigh*
Pick up, roll and wring the inner, middle and outer thigh muscles to bring the deeper toxins to the surface and to eliminate fatty deposits.

4 *Effleuraging the thigh*
Effleurage the thigh to eliminate further toxins.

5 *Patella*
Work all around the patella (knee cap) using small circular friction movements (see Figure 4.17).

6 *Effleuraging the lower leg*
Effleurage the lower half of the leg with cupped hands from ankle to knee. Use less pressure on this bony, more delicate area than you did on the thigh.

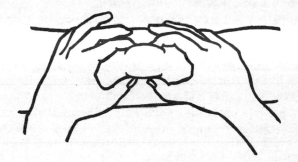

figure 4.17   use small circular movements around the patella (knee cap)

7 *Petrissaging the lower leg*
Gently petrissage along the outside of the tibialis anterior muscle of the lower leg. You can see this muscle easily if the receiver pulls his or her foot back.

8 *Effleuraging the leg*
Effleurage the entire leg.

9 *Tapotement*
Cup and hack the thigh **only**. Never perform tapotement movements over the bony areas of the lower leg.

10 *Completion*
Effleurage the entire leg, gradually decreasing the pressure with each movement.

Repeat on the other leg

Abdomen

Four pairs of muscles form the strong anterior wall of the abdomen. When they contract they compress the abdomen – thus they help in functions such as defecation, childbirth, forced expiration and so on. They also have a very important postural function in that they pull the front of the pelvis upwards, flattening the lumbar curve of the spine. If these muscles lose their tone then the abdomen protrudes.

The abdomen is an often neglected area of the body as far as massage is concerned. Remember when massaging the abdomen that you are working on muscles and viscera. The benefits that can be derived from abdominal massage are considerable.

The benefits of abdominal massage

- Constipation, bloatedness and flatulence can be relieved. If the problem is chronic then diet and nutrition should be altered.
- After an operation (e.g. Caesarean or appendix), once scar tissue has begun to heal, massage will help to prevent adhesion formation and scar contractures.
- If there is visceroptosis (prolapse of the viscera) where the contents of the abdomen drop to a lower level, massage will help if it is combined with exercise, provided that there is still some tone left in the muscles. If muscle tone is restored to the outer wall by massage then the internal organs may be held in a normal position. Visceroptosis may occur due to incorrect posture, abdominal surgery, inadequate support or insufficient muscle toning after childbirth.

But do not:

- massage over **recent** scar tissue until it has healed and only then with the permission of a doctor (once healing is established massage is excellent for preventing adhesions)
- massage where there is inflammation of any organs in the abdomen (e.g. gastritis, appendicitis, colitis)
- massage the abdomen within one hour of a heavy meal
- use heavy pressure over the abdomen during pregnancy
- use heavy pressure during the first few days of menstruation if it is uncomfortable
- encourage the receiver to talk or laugh during the abdominal massage because the muscles tighten making treatment impossible
- massage the abdomen if the bladder is full (suggest a visit to the lavatory prior to a treatment).

The massage

1 Circular effleurage (two handed)
Make sure you are positioned on the receiver's right-hand side when you start the massage so that you are able to follow the colon in the appropriate direction. Place both your hands on the receiver's navel, one hand on top of the other, and move in a

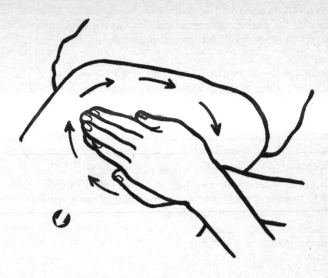

figure 4.21   double-handed effleurage of the abdomen

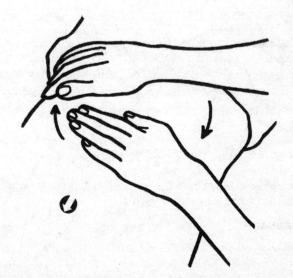

figure 4.22   circular effleurage of the abdomen, one hand following the other

clockwise direction with a circular movement. Gradually increase the size of the circles until the entire abdomen is covered. Use gentle pressure at first, gradually increasing the depth of the strokes as the receiver relaxes.

2 *Circular effleurage (one handed)*
Moving in a clockwise direction, circle around the abdomen with one hand following behind the other (see Figure 4.21).

3 *Colon massage*
To treat the colon, begin at the bottom right-hand side of the abdomen. With the flat surface of the three middle fingers of one hand work around the colon in a clockwise direction using small circular friction movements (see Figure 4.23). The colon massage begins at the **caecum,** up the **ascending colon** to the **hepatic flexure,** across the **transverse colon** to the **splenic flexure** and down the **descending colon** to the **sigmoid colon.** Slide your hand across the abdomen to the starting position using no pressure. Repeat several times.

4 *Circular effleurage (two handed)*
Repeat the clockwise circular stroking, working smoothly with one hand following the other.

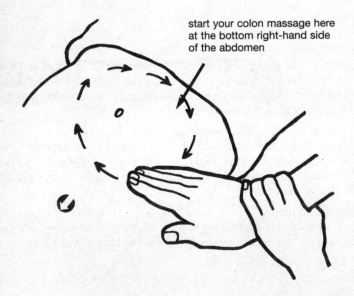

start your colon massage here at the bottom right-hand side of the abdomen

figure 4.23 gently massage the colon

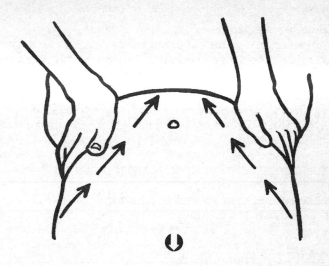

figure 4.24 drain the abdomen

5 *Draining the abdomen (one side)*
Using both hands, one on top of the other, reach across to the receiver's far side underneath the abdomen and pull upwards and then downwards towards the bladder. Repeat on the other side of the abdomen.

6 *Draining the abdomen (both sides)*
Reach under the receiver's abdomen so that your fingers are touching each other (waistline permitting). Pull both hands at the same time upwards and downwards towards the bladder (see Figure 4.24).

7 *Petrissaging*
Pick up and roll and wring the waist and hip area opposite you. Repeat on the other side of the waist and hip area.

8 *Circular effleurage*
Effleurage the entire abdomen with one hand following after the other.

9 *Tapotement*
Reaching over the opposite side, gently cup and hack the waist and hip area to increase muscular tone and to break down fatty deposits.

10 *Rocking the pelvis*
Using your palms, place one hand on each side of the receiver's pelvis. Rock gently and slowly. This movement loosens the pelvic area and encourages the whole body to relax.

11 *Completion*
Repeat the clockwise effleurage with one hand following the other. Gradually decrease the pressure and let your hands come to rest on the navel.

Arm and hand

The benefits of arm and hand massage
Our arms and hands are in constant use in our everyday activities in the home, at work and in our leisure pursuits. It is not surprising that they are prone to so many injuries. Massage can afford a great deal of relief.

But do not:
- work over recent fractures
- massage directly over areas of inflammation such as swollen joints
- massage directly over **recent** scar tissue
- massage infectious skin conditions
- use heavy pressure where the skin is thin or bruises easily
- use heavy pressure on the delicate area at the front of the elbow joint (cubital fossa).

The massage
1 *Effleuraging the arm*
Position yourself beside the receiver and effleurage the entire arm from the wrist to the shoulder. You may perform this effleurage in two ways (see Figure 4.18):

- support the arm carefully underneath with one hand as you effleurage (if necessary you may use a pillow too)
- use one hand to 'shake hands' with the receiver and the other to effleurage.

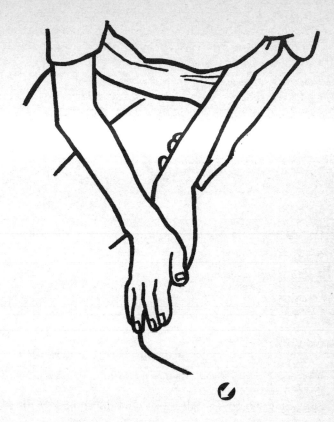

figure 4.18 effleurage the whole arm

2 *Friction the shoulder*
To loosen and mobilize the shoulder joint use slow circular friction movements around the front, top and back of the shoulder joint.

3 *Petrissaging the upper arm*
Bend the receiver's arm and place the forearm across the body so that it is resting and supported on the receiver's upper abdomen. Pick up, roll and wring the biceps and triceps muscles of the upper arm firmly and rhythmically (see Figure 4.19).

4 *Friction the elbow*
Supporting the arm use the circular friction movements around the elbow joint to relieve pain and stiffness. If there is any sensitivity then decrease your pressure circles.

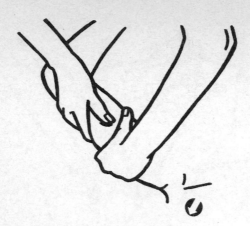

figure 4.19   wring the muscles of the upper arm

5 *Effleuraging the arm*

Effleurage the entire arm to encourage any toxins that have been released to move towards the axillary lymph glands in the armpit.

6 *Effleuraging the forearm*

With the receiver's upper arm down and the forearm lifted, effleurage firmly from the wrist to the elbow (see Figure 4.20).

7 *Friction the wrist joint*

Using your thumbs, friction into the carpal bones of the wrist.

8 *Mobilizing the wrist*

Interlace your fingers with the receiver's fingers (if the size of hands is compatible) and bend the wrist slowly, gently and carefully backwards and forwards, side to side and circumduct the wrist clockwise and anticlockwise. This is excellent exercise for the wrist flexors and extensors.

9 *Friction the hand*

Friction with your thumbs into the palm of the receiver's hand and also into the back of the hand. This will loosen the metacarpals.

10 *Mobilizing the fingers*

To work the 14 phalanges, gently and slowly squeeze and stretch each finger individually. With your thumb and index finger friction the phalanges. Flex and extend each phalange – remember there are two in the thumb joint and three in the fingers. Circumduct each finger individually clockwise and anticlockwise.

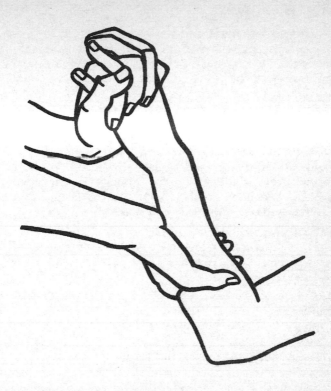

figure 4.20   effleurage the forearms from wrist to elbow

11 *Effleuraging the arm*
Effleurage the entire arm with pressure, as always, up the arm towards the heart and the axilliary lymph glands. Glide gently back, gradually decreasing the pressure with each movement.

12 *Completion*
On the final stroke, clasp the receiver's hand between the palms of your hands and squeeze gently.

Repeat on the other arm

Chest and neck

The benefits of chest and neck massage

The chest area plays a vital role in the breathing process. If it is constricted by tension, the ribcage is unable to expand and contract as we breathe in and breathe out. Excessive tightness in the chest can even lead to conditions such as panic attacks, hyperventilation (over-breathing) and other anxiety states where an individual may mistakenly believe that he or she is experiencing a heart attack. Massage of the chest area enables us to breathe more deeply and evenly and also aids the elimination of toxins and mucus. Emotional problems may often be stored in the chest area – in our everyday language we have the expression 'get if off your chest'. Massage encourages us to release these bottled-up emotions.

The neck area is vulnerable to physical and emotional stress and tension. Contraction in the neck muscles is a major contributory factor to headaches. Massage is an excellent way of relieving this tension.

But do not:

- apply heavy pressure to the delicate area of the chest and neck
- massage inflamed or sensitive areas
- massage infectious skin conditions
- work directly over **recent** scar tissue, open wounds or **recent** fractures
- massage over lumps: these should be checked by a doctor.

The massage

1 *Effleuraging the chest*

Position yourself at the receiver's head and place your hands in the centre of the chest just below the collar bones. Relax your fingers and with the back of both hands, effleurage gently outwards towards the armpits (see Figure 4.25). As you reach the shoulders turn your hands over and use the palms to stroke and direct the lymph into the axillary glands under the arms. Stroke back with no pressure to the starting position. Repeat several times.

2 *Friction the chest*

Start in the centre of the receiver's chest below the clavicles. Make gentle circular friction movements with your thumbs or fingers, working towards and around the front of the shoulders.

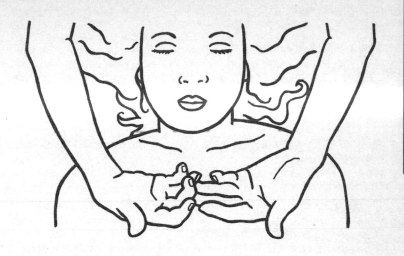

figure 4.25 effleurage across the upper chest

3 *Petrissaging the chest*
With alternate hands pick up, squeeze and wring the fleshy area in front of the receiver's armpit. Work with both hands on one side and then slide the hands across the body and repeat on the opposite side. These movements on the pectoral muscles help to release further tension in the chest.

4 *Stretching the chest and shoulder muscles*
Cup your hands around the top of both shoulders and gently push the shoulders down towards the feet. Repeat several times.

Move your hands so that they cup the front of the shoulders, and with straight arms, press down. Hold this position for approximately five seconds and release slowly. Repeat several times.

5 *Releasing the neck*
Reach under the neck with both hands so that your fingertips touch and gently stroke, pulling up and towards you.

6 *Side stroking*
Turn the head to one side. Place one hand on the forehead and stroke the other hand from the ear, down the side of the neck and over the shoulder. Repeat on the other side of the neck.

7 *Friction the skull*
With the head straight, feel the base of the skull with the fingers of both hands. Make circular friction movements around the base of the skull.

8 *Stretching the neck*
Cup both your hands under the back of the head, with the fingers at the base of the skull. Pull gently and slowly towards you as you lean backwards, thus using your own body weight to traction the neck. Never jerk or pull the neck suddenly.

9 *Completion*
Rest your cupped hands gently on the forehead to relax and soothe the receiver.

Face

The benefits of face massage

Massage treatment of the face is an effective way to relieve headaches of all descriptions, whether caused by stress, sinus congestion, menstrual or digestive problems. As the circulation to the face is improved, the complexion is rejuvenated and takes on a healthy glow. Some individuals opt for regular facial massage in preference to a face lift as the effects are so noticeable. People can look years younger.

But do not:

- massage over contact lenses
- work on inflamed or swollen areas
- massage over **recent** scar tissue
- massage over infectious skin conditions or areas of infection such as spots or boils
- use heavy pressure on the delicate area of the face.

The massage

1 *Effleuraging the forehead*
Stroke out across the forehead using the relaxed fingertips of the back of your hands (see Figure 4.26). Let your hands glide back with no pressure.

2 *Effleuraging the cheeks*
Stroke outwards across the cheeks towards the ears.

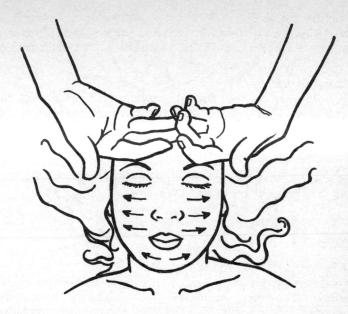

figure 4.26 effleurage the forehead, cheels and chin

3 *Effleuraging the chin*
Stroke outwards across the chin and jaw and continue to effleurage down the neck towards the shoulder.

4 *Working the forehead in strips*
Place both thumbs in the centre of the receiver's forehead just above the eyebrows with your fingers around the sides of the head. Slowly but firmly press and release at intervals, working outwards in a row. Work up the forehead in strips covering the whole forehead as far as the hairline.

5 *Decongesting the cheek bones*
Start under the eyes, and with your thumbs stroke outwards across the cheeks. Cover the whole of the cheek area in horizontal strips, and as you reach the ears massage them using your thumbs and first two fingers. Stretch and release the ears gently.

6 *Decongesting the chin*
Begin just under the mouth, and with your thumbs press outwards. Cover the entire chin and jaw area, again working in horizontal strips.

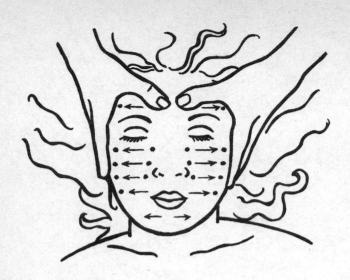

figure 4.27   work across the face in strips using pressure points

7 Unblocking the nasal passages
Using both thumbs stroke down the sides of the nose.

8 Releasing the scalp tension
Using your fingertips, massage the hairline from the top of the forehead around to the base of the skull with deep circular friction movements. Perform these movements firmly and slowly.

9 Completion
Stroke the hair gently from the roots to the tips to release the last remaining tension. Gradually allow your hands to come to rest on the temples.

At the end of the treatment wash your hands throughly under cold, running water to cleanse yourself physically and psychically.

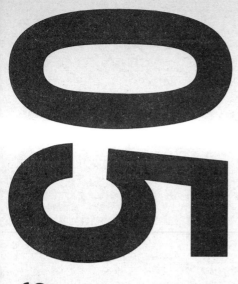

05

self-massage

Self massage is a wonderful way to soothe away stress and tension and to treat common disorders such as tired legs and feet, back pain, colon problems, headaches and so on. It also has the advantage that you can perform it as often as you wish at almost any time and place.

Ideally you should massage yourself at least once a week. If you are experiencing discomfort such as low back pain or a sore neck then massage the affected area daily. You will be amazed at the relief.

As you perform the massage movements on yourself, discover which ones feel particularly good. As you practice on yourself you will become more proficient at massaging others and as a bonus your health will improve.

Legs

Massage will help to relieve your tired and achy legs at the end of the day. You can prevent varicose veins, improve circulation, reduce swelling and improve the appearance of unsightly cellulite.

A simple leg massage prior to or after exercise is a wonderful way of preventing injuries and relieving stiffness.

Position for massage

Sitting down on the floor or on a bed with one leg stretched out straight in front of you and the other leg bent with the foot flat on the ground.

1 *Calf muscles – effleurage*

Effleurage from your heel to the back of your knee using one or both hands (see Figure 5.1). Place both hands at the front of the leg and stroke upwards, using your fingers with the pressure reinforced by your overlying hand.

2 *Calf muscles – petrissage*

Keeping your knee bent, work on your calf muscles at the back of your leg. Pick up, roll and wring this area.

3 *Achilles tendon – friction*

With your fingers and thumbs apply deep friction to your Achilles tendon.

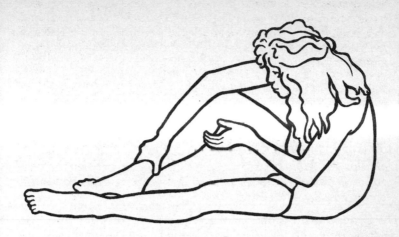

figure 5.1 effleurage the calf

4 *Knee – friction*
Place the pads of both thumbs just below the knee and use small circular friction movements all around the patella. These movements will help to improve and maintain mobility of your knee joint.

5 *Thigh – effleurage*
Stroke firmly up from the knee towards the groin. Ensure that you effleurage all aspects of the thigh.

6 *Thigh – petrissage*
Squeeze and wring the inner, middle and outer thigh muscles. This can help to break down fatty deposits and if performed daily may greatly improve the shape of your thighs! If you wish to pay extra attention to certain areas then make your hands into loose fists and perform circular movements with your knuckles.

7 *Cellulite buster!*
Lightly clench your fists and bring them down onto any areas of cellulite in quick succession.

Finish with effleurage.

Feet

Massage of the feet is not only a very pleasurable and relaxing experience but also helps to improve the health of the entire body. According to reflexology the feet are a mirror of the body and by massaging the feet you are treating all the organs, glands and structures of the body.

Position for massage

Sitting down on the floor, on a bed or a chair. Bend the knee and place the foot to be treated onto the opposite thigh.

1 Foot – *effleurage*

With one hand under the sole of the foot and the other on the top stroke firmly upwards.

2 Foot – *friction sole*

Use both thumbs to make small circular movements all over the sole of the foot. This opens up and loosens the tendons and muscles of the foot.

3 Ankle – *friction and move*

Use your thumbs or fingertips to make circular movements all around the ankle joint. Gently and slowly circle your ankle both clockwise and anti-clockwise.

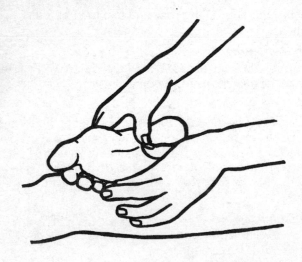

figure 5.2   place the foot to be treated on the opposite thigh

4 *Toes – friction and move*
Using your thumb and index finger, friction the toe joints both top and bottom to loosen them. Then slowly stretch and move each of them both clockwise and anti-clockwise.

Neck and shoulders

Tightness in the neck and shoulders is an extremely common symptom of stress and often gives rise to headaches. These simple techniques can help to break down the numerous knots and nodules that arise and will improve neck mobility enormously. Try these movements when you feel stressed or to prevent headaches from occurring.

Position for massage
Sitting on a chair, bed or the floor with both feet flat on the ground.

1 *Neck – effleurage*
Relax your neck forwards and place your hands behind your head, fingertips touching or slightly overlapping. Apply deep, downwards effleurage movements down the neck.

2 *Neck – friction*
Apply small circular friction movements to the base of your skull using your fingertips.

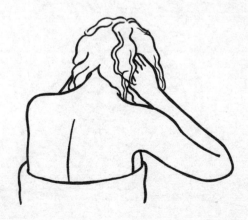

figure 5.3   friction to the base of the skull

3 *Shoulders – effleurage*

To massage your right shoulder reach across the front of your chest and place your left hand at the base of the skull and stroke firmly down the side of the neck and over your shoulder. Repeat on the other shoulder.

4 *Shoulders – pick up and squeeze*

Reach across the front of your chest again and squeeze and release the muscles on top of the other shoulder picking up as much flesh as possible.

Repeat steps 3 and 4 on the other shoulder.

5 *Scapulae – friction*

Reach across the front of your body with your right hand to touch your left shoulder blade at the back of your body (See Figure 5.4. Use your fingertips to apply deep pressure to any knots or nodules.

Repeat on the other scapula.

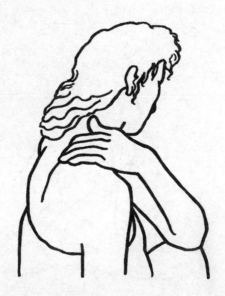

figure 5.4 friction of the scapula

Back

This is a difficult area to reach without stretching, but it is worth persevering for the benefits you will derive.

Most of you will suffer from back pain at least once in your lifetime. Self-massage of the back can dramatically reduce back pain. If you are prone to back problems perform this routine daily.

Position for massage

Sit down on the floor, on a stool or on a bed.

1 Press your thumbs into the dimples on either side of your spine. Perform circular friction movements working up your back slowly and deeply travelling as far up as you can. (See Figure 5.5). Search out the knots and nodules in the erector spinae muscle group, and when you encounter them, apply firmer pressure to break them down. If you find it difficult to use your thumbs, then use the pads of several of your fingers instead.

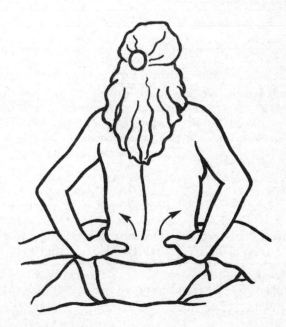

figure 5.5 friction the back

2 Place your hands behind your back, one flat palm either side of your spine. Firmly effleurage down your back. Perform this movement slowly to relax and soothe or quickly to stimulate and invigorate. This movement may also be performed using lightly clenched fists.

3 Place both hands in the middle of your lower back, fingertips pointing downwards. Make large outward circles with both hands simultaneously to loosen and decongest the lumbar area and buttocks. If you need a deeper treatment, use the knuckles of your fists on the gluteal muscles and the iliac crest.

Abdomen

Abdominal massage will encourage regular bowel movements, relieve the discomfort of abdominal bloating and aid the digestion, absorption and elimination of food. After abdominal surgery such as a caesarean or an appendectomy, once the scar tissue has healed massage helps to prevent the formation of adhesions and speeds up recovery. If performed daily muscle tone will also be improved.

Position for massage
Lying down on your back with your knees bent up and your feet apart so that your abdominal muscles are completely relaxed.

1 Abdomen – circular effleurage
Place your hands flat down, one on top of the other on your navel. Make large slow circular movements, proceeding in a clockwise direction. These strokes will help to relieve any emotional trauma stored in your abdomen.

2 Colon – friction
To encourage regular bowel movements, friction your colon gently with the three middle fingers of your hand. Start at the bottom right hand side of your abdomen working up the ascending colon. Friction across the abdomen to stimulate the transverse colon. To complete your colon massage, work down the descending colon to the left hand side of your abdomen.

3 Abdomen – tapotement
To stimulate digestion and improve muscle tone, perform very gentle cupping.

Arm and hand

Our arms, wrists and hands are used constantly in our daily activities. Aches and pains in the arms and hands are often caused by repetitive movements, although they may be the result of a neck problem. Massage of these areas is essential to promote strength and mobility and is particularly beneficial to people who use their hands and arms extensively in the course of their work – for example individuals who use computer keyboards, gardeners and hairdressers. Treatment is also essential for sports people for preventing injuries from occurring. According to hand reflexology all the parts of the body are mirrored in miniature on the hands. For further information please refer to my other book in the series *Teach Yourself Hand Reflexology*.

Position for massage

Sitting down on the floor, bed or a chair. Rest your hand gently on your lap.

1 *Arm – effleurage*

Place the palm of your hand on your wrist and effleurage the whole arm up to the shoulder.

2 *Upper arm – effleurage*

Apply deep stroking to the flexor muscles on the front of your upper arm (biceps, brachialis) and the extensor muscles (triceps) on the back of your upper arm. Always work up your arm trying to move the lymph up the axillary glands in your armpit.

3 *Upper arm – petrissage*

Squeeze and wring the muscles of your upper arm to break down any adhesions and to bring the deeper toxins to the surface.

4 *Lower arm – deep stroking*

With your elbow flexed and the tip of your elbow resting on your abdomen to encourage drainage, apply deep downward longitudinal stroking to the flexor and extensor muscles of your lower arm.

5 *Wrist – loosen and move*

Use your thumb and fingertips to gently friction all around the wrist joint. After these loosening movements interlock your fingers and circle the wrist clockwise and anti-clockwise.

6 *Palm – circular kneading*

With a clenched fist, work into the palm of your hand with circular movements to loosen up the muscles, tendons and joints.

7 *Fingers and thumb – loosen and move*

Using your thumb and index finger gently stretch each finger and thumb. Then circle each one individually. These movements will ease rheumatic complaints and arthritis.

Face and scalp

Face and scalp massage is a wonderful way to relax and unwind, completely banishing tiredness and anxiety, relieving headaches and clearing sinuses. Over a period of time, as circulation and drainage is stimulated, you will also notice improvements in your complexion and fine wrinkles may disappear.

Position for massage

Lying down on the floor or bed or sitting up on a chair if you prefer.

1 *Face effleurage*

Place both hands palms down on your forehead with your fingertips facing each other. Stroke across your forehead. Repeat this outward movement, stroking across your cheeks and across your chin.

2 *Eyes – stroking*

Use your index or your index and middle fingers to effleurage very gently outwards underneath each eye. Take great care, as this is a very delicate area. These movements will help to relieve puffiness and to prevent and reduce fine lines.

3 *Chin and jaw – toning*

Pinch all along your jaw line using your thumbs and index finger to help prevent a double chin.

4 *Eyebrows – toning*

Starting at the inside of your eyebrows, pinch your brow bone until you reach the end of your eyebrow. Repeat each movement several times.

5 *Mouth – friction*

Make a large 'O' with your mouth. Using your index and middle fingers apply small circular friction movements around your mouth. These movements may help to stop fine wrinkles appearing.

6 Scalp – friction

With your fingertips, use small rotary movements covering your entire scalp. These movements will remove tension from your scalp and by aiding circulation can also make your hair healthier.

7 Completion

To finish your massage programme, place the heels of your hands over your eyes. Hold your hands there for a few seconds allowing your eyes to relax completely in darkness as you gently remove your hands. You will feel revitalized and refreshed.

If you have enjoyed massaging the face and scalp you may like to refer to my other book in this series *Teach Yourself Indian Head Massage*.

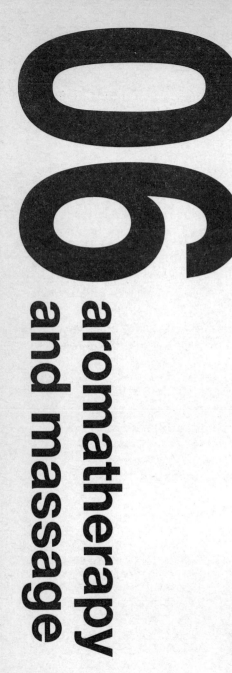

06

aromatherapy and massage

In this chapter you will learn:
- how to make up a blend using essential oils
- the properties and effects of 16 common essential oils.

The healing art of aromatherapy – the use of pure essential oils to maintain physical, mental and spiritual health – is a wonderful way of enhancing the therapeutic effects of your massage.

This chapter is not intended to be a complete guide to aromatherapy but it will cover some of the most versatile essential oils. There are, in fact, more than 200 plants from which essential oils are extracted. For further information please refer to my other book in this series *Teach Yourself Aromatherapy*.

Essential oils

Blending

Essential oils are extremely concentrated. Always blend them with a suitable carrier oil in the appropriate dilution when using them for massage (see pages 12–15). A few essential oils may be used undiluted to treat injuries such as wasp stings, cuts or burns.

The essential oil content in a blend should usually be between 1 per cent and 3 per cent. Use the following as a rough guideline:

   5 ml carrier oil = 1 teaspoon
   10 ml carrier oil = 1 dessertspoon
   15 ml carrier oil = 1 tablespoon

   Add 1–2 drops of pure essential oil to 5 ml of carrier oil
   Add 3–4 drops of pure essential oil to 10 ml of carrier oil
   Add 5 drops of pure essential oil to 15 ml of carrier oil
   Add 6–8 drops of pure essential oil to 20 ml of carrier oil

A full body massage will require approximately 20 ml of oil.

Storage of essential oils

Essential oils should always be stored in dark coloured rather than clear glass bottles as the oils deteriorate in sunlight. Amber coloured bottles are by far the best. Essential oils are volatile, so replace the caps immediately after use otherwise the oils will gradually evaporate. Always keep essential oils at an even temperature – avoid direct sunlight and shelves on radiators.

If you keep pure essential oils in amber glass bottles in a cool place, they should have a shelf life of approximately two to three years. Citrus essential oils have the shortest shelf life. Once an essential oil has been diluted in a carrier oil or cream, it will keep for only a few months.

Purchasing

It is important to buy only pure essential oils if you want to achieve the best results. Synthetic and adulterated oils carry with them the risk of unpleasant and harmful side effects. Essential oils may be adulterated by adding alcohol, synthetic products or cheaper essential oils. Make sure you buy **pure** essential oils, not oils that have already been diluted in a carrier oil. (See 'Useful Addresses'.)

Massage with essential oils

Massage with essential oils is an extremely powerful method of application. The minute molecules of essential oil penetrate the skin and can reach the bloodstream and lymph. Aromatherapy massage is the only treatment technique discussed in this book. Other methods include inhalations, baths, foot and hand baths, showers, saunas, compresses, gargles and mouthwashes. For further information please refer to *Teach Yourself Aromatherapy*.

I have chosen 16 of the most common essential oils used in aromatherapy today with particular emphasis on their uses and indications. If medical conditions are severe and persistent, consult a qualified medical practitioner before treatment.

Bergamot

Latin name   *Citrus bergamia*   Keywords   Antidepressant
Family   RUTACEAE   Antiseptic
                                              Balancing
                                              Uplifting

Principal properties and effects

- An invaluable oil for stress, anxiety and depression possessing an uplifting yet sedative quality.
- Helpful for infections of the urinary tract, vaginal infections, itching and thrush.
- Beneficial for the digestive system. Relieves indigestion, flatulence and loss of appetite as in anorexia.
- Excellent for infections of the respiratory system including sore throats, tonsillitis and bronchitis.
- Useful for the skin as an antiseptic for acne, seborrhea of the skin and scalp. Also for infectious conditions such as chicken pox and shingles.

Special precautions

Avoid strong sunlight after use as bergamot increases the photo-sensitivity of the skin due to the chemical bergapten.

Chamomile (ROMAN)

Latin name	*Anthemis nobilis*	Keywords	Balancing
Family	COMPOSITAE/		Calming
	ASTERACEAE		Redness and irritation
			Soothing

Principal properties and effects

- Particularly suitable for use with infants and sensitive individuals, asthma, colic, infections, skin problems and temper tantrums.
- Excellent for inflammatory disorders as the essential oil contains the powerful anti-inflammatory agent azulene formed during distillation – colitis, gastritis and dermatitis.
- Beneficial for skin care, soothing allergic and hypersensitive skin, boils, burns and inflamed wounds. Helpful for eczema and dry itchy skin.
- Its analgesic action relieves aches and pains whether in muscles, joints or organs – backache, earache, headache, stomach ache, toothache.
- Renowned for its soothing effects on the nervous system promoting relaxation and deep sleep (chamomile tea is a popular infusion for relieving insomnia). Dispels anger, anxiety, fear and tension.
- Popular for menstrual disorders – dysmenorrhoea, menopause, menorrhagia, pre-menstrual syndrome. It balances the hormones, eases period pain, regulates the menstrual cycle and relieves anger and irritability.
- Useful for boosting the immune system. It stimulates the leucocytes (white blood cells) and thus reduces the frequency and severity of infections.

Special precautions

None! Roman chamomile is an extremely safe oil.

Cypress

Latin name *Cupressus sempervirens* Keywords Astringent
Family   CUPRESSACEAE   Fluid reducing
                                         Restorative

Principal properties and effects

- Helpful whenever there is excessive fluid – oedema, sweating (particularly of the feet), bedwetting.
- Renowned for regulating the menstrual cycle and for relieving menstrual problems, particularly PMS (pre-menstrual syndrome) and the hot flushes, hormonal imbalances, irritability and depression of the menopause.
- Balances oily skin, puffiness, cellulite.
- Its comforting and restorative properties help to ease grief. Cypress alleviates nervous tension and stress-related conditions.
- Excellent for varicose veins due to its vasoconstricting effect. Use gentle effleurage only.

Special precautions

None! Cypress is non-irritant, non-sensitizing and non-toxic.

Eucalyptus

Latin name *Eucalyptus globulus* Keywords Analgesic
Family   MYRTACEAE   (pain relieving)
                                        Antiseptic
                                        Expectorant
                                         (clears out
                                             mucus)
                                        Stimulant

Principal properties and effects

- Excellent as an inhalant and chest rub for all respiratory disorders – asthma, catarrh, colds, coughs, sinusitis and throat infections.
- Provides pain relief for arthritis, muscular aches and pains and rheumatism.
- Powerful essential oil for stimulating the brain and aiding concentration.
- Effective for all types of fever and infectious illnesses.

Special precautions

- Store away from homoeopathic medications.
- Do not use on babies and young children.

Frankincense

Latin name *Boswellia carterii*
Family   BURSERACEAE

Keywords Expectorant
         Elevating
         Haunting
         Healing
         Rejuvenating

Principal properties and effects

- Engenders an elevating yet soothing effect on the emotions allowing past traumas and anxiety to fade away.
- Encourages the breath to slow down and deepen making it ideal for asthma and all respiratory disorders especially when linked with stress. Particularly conducive to prayer and meditation.
- An excellent remedy for all skin care. Frankincense rejuvenates mature and ageing skin, toning and smoothing out the wrinkles. Heals ulcers and wounds.

Special precautions

None.

Geranium

Latin name *Pelargonium graveolens*
Family   GERANIACEAE

Keywords Antidepressant
         Balancing
         Healing
         Uplifting

Principal properties and effects

- Particularly beneficial for the nervous system, dispelling anxiety states and depression and uplifting the spirit.
- Highly effective for the menopause and PMS balancing the hormones, reducing fluid and alleviating tension.
- Stimulates the lymphatic system encouraging the elimination of toxins.

- Excellent for all skin types due to its ability to balance sebum. Useful for congested, dry, inflamed, oily or combination skin, burns, eczema, herpes and wounds.

Special precautions

None.

Jasmine

Latin name *Jasminum officinale*
Family OLEACEAE

Keywords Aphrodisiac
Euphoric
Healing
Strengthening

Principal properties and effects

Jasmine is often referred to as the 'King of essential oils' and is frequently adulterated due to its high price.

- Invaluable for treating depression, inducing feelings of optimism, confidence and euphoria. Useful for apathy and indifference.
- Highly effective in childbirth, promoting the contractions yet inducing relaxation and relieving the pain. It promotes the flow of breast milk after the birth and prevents post-natal depression.
- A renowned aphrodisiac, jasmine alleviates premature ejaculation, frigidity and impotence. It strengthens the male sex organs and increases the sperm count.
- Beneficial for all skin types especially dry, sensitive skin. Useful for stretchmarks and scars and for increasing the elasticity of the skin.

Special precautions

Do not take internally.

Juniper

Latin name *Juniperus communis*
Family CUPRESSACEAE

Keywords Antiseptic
Detoxifying
Fluid reducing
Purifying

Principal properties and effects

- A classic remedy for urinary infections such as cystitis. Excellent for relieving fluid retention and for those who have difficulty in passing urine.
- Renowned for its detoxifying and purifying ability, juniper clears waste from the body as well as from the mind. Helpful for obesity, and after too much rich food and alcohol. An ideal oil for emotional depletion clearing and strengthening the mind.
- Effective for arthritis, gout and rheumatic disorders stimulating the elimination of uric acid and other toxins.
- Indicated for acne, blocked pores, oily and congested skin, purifying and encouraging detoxification.

Special precautions

- Avoid during pregnancy.
- Do not use excessively where there is inflammation of the kidneys.

Lavender

Latin name	*Lavandula officinalis/ vera/angustifolia*	Keywords	Analgesic
Family	LAMIACEAE (or Labiatae)		Antidepressant
			Balancing
			Healing
			Rejuvenating
			Soothing

Principal properties and effects

Lavender is one of the most popular and versatile essential oils used in aromatherapy. Its aroma is familiar to almost everyone – well established as a remedy.

- Highly recommended for the nervous system relieving depression, anxiety and insomnia. Balances mood swings and soothes anger, frustration and irritability. Useful for shock.
- Helpful for high blood pressure, palpitations and other cardiac disorders.
- Invaluable for pain relief in conditions such as arthritis, lumbago, rheumatism, sprains and strains.

- Renowned as an immune system booster, lavender is recommended for all infections and viruses, catarrh, colds and throat disorders.
- Excellent for all skin care due to its powers of rejuvenation and balancing effects. Helps to heal burns, sunburn, acne, boils, bruises, eczema, psoriasis and wounds and sores of all descriptions.

Special precautions

None. A gentle essential oil suitable for all ages from babies to the elderly.

Lemon

Latin name *Citrus limonum*   Keywords Alkaline
Family   RUTACEAE   Antiseptic
                                        Purifying
                                        Revitalising
                                        Stimulant

Principal properties and effects

- Highly recommended for the digestive system, particularly for counteracting acidity.
- Indicated for all infectious diseases, lemon boosts the immune system, reduces high temperatures and restores vitality, accelerating recovery time.
- Popular for skin care. Its cleansing action makes it suitable for oily skin (and hair), cuts and infected wounds, warts and varrucae.
- Stimulating for the circulatory system, liquefying the blood. Helpful for varicose veins (together with cypress) – gentle effleurage only.

Special precautions

Avoid strong sunlight immediately after treatment.

Neroli (Orange blossom)

Latin name *Citrus aurantium* Keywords Antidepressant
                                          Aphrodisiac
Family   RUTACEAE   Rejuvenative
                                          Tranquillising

Principal properties and effects

- Invaluable for all nervous problems, neroli is one of the most effective antidepressant/sedative oils. Relieves chronic or short-term anxiety, soothes hysteria and shock and induces sleep. Suitable for individuals with addictions.
- Effective for colic, colitis, diarrhoea and nervous indigestion.
- Recommended for reducing scarring and the prevention of stretchmarks. Neroli is beneficial for all skin types, encouraging the regeneration of skin cells, particularly dry, mature and sensitive skin.
- Due to its aphrodisiac properties, effective for sexual problems such as impotence and frigidity.

Special precautions

None. A very gentle oil.

Peppermint

Latin name *Mentha piperita* Keywords Analgesic
Family   LAMIACEAE   Cooling
            (or Labiatae)   Digestive
                                         Pain relieving
                                         Stimulating

Principal properties and effects

- Exerts a powerful effect on the digestive system. Recommended for nausea and vomiting (travel sickness), diarrhoea and constipation. Relieves pain and spasm in the stomach and colon.
- Its pain relieving properties make it invaluable for headaches and migraine, particularly if related to digestion. Highly effective for reducing muscular aches, neuralgia and rheumatism.

- Useful for stimulating the mind, eliminating mental fatigue and encouraging clarity of thought.
- Peppermint cools down sunburn and inflammation. Helpful for toxic congested skin, acne and oily skin.

Special precautions

- Store away from homoeopathic medications.
- Take care with sensitive skins – use in low concentrations.
- Avoid when breast-feeding as it discourages the flow of breast milk.
- Do not use on babies and young children.

Rose

Latin name	*Rosa centifolia/ damascena*	Keywords	Antidepressant Aphrodisiac
Family	ROSACEAE		Lingering and loving Rejuvenating

Principal properties and effects

- The exquisite, luxurious aroma of rose has a profound effect on the emotions, filling the heart with love and alleviating depression, grief, jealousy, resentment, shock and tension.
- An invaluable oil for all female problems, regulating the menstrual cycle and cleansing and toning the womb. Helpful for PMS and the menopause. Recommended for frigidity, impotence and other sexual difficulties.
- Excellent for all types of skin, particularly dry, mature and sensitive skin. Reduces broken thread veins.

Special precautions

None. Invaluable for women and gentle enough for use on children.

Rosemary

Latin name	*Rosmarinus officinalis*	Keywords	Analgesic
Family	LAMIACEAE (or Labiatae)		Detoxifying Fluid reducing Restorative Stimulating

Principal properties and effects

- An invaluable restorative for loss of function, reviving muscles, limbs, memory, hair, smell and so forth.
- Highly recommended for pain relief in muscles and joints, easing arthritis, gout, rheumatism and stiff, overworked muscles.
- Activates and enlivens the brain, clearing the head and reducing mental fatigue.
- Beneficial for a wide range of digestive complaints where detoxification is required as with constipation, flatulence and liver congestion.
- Useful for combating fluid retention and lymphatic congestion. Effective for cellulite and obesity.
- Beneficial for the hair and scalp, encouraging hair growth and alleviating dandruff.

Special precautions

Do not use excessively in pregnancy or in cases of epilepsy.

Sandalwood

Latin name	*Santalum album*	Keywords	Aphrodisiac
Family	SANTALACEAE		Healing
			Relaxing
			Uplifting

Principal properties and effects

- Well known for its balancing effects on the nervous system, gently soothing away anxiety and tension. Sandalwood engenders feelings of peace and tranquillity.
- Particularly valuable for urinary infections alleviating cystitis and vaginal discharges of all kinds.
- Helpful for sexual problems such as impotence and frigidity.
- Used extensively for skin complaints, sandalwood is particularly beneficial for dry, cracked, chapped or dehydrated skin. When blended with a carrier oil it makes an excellent aftershave.

Special precautions

None.

Tea tree

Latin name *Melaleuca alternifolia* Keywords Antiseptic
Family MYRTACEAE Antifungal
Anti-infectious
Stimulating

Principal properties and effects

- Renowned for its remarkable activity against bacteria, fungi and viruses and as a powerful immuno-stimulant, tea tree is a must for the first aid kit in every household. Particularly useful for repeated infections, pre- and post-operatively and for post-viral syndromes such as ME (*myalgic encephalomyelitis*). Invaluable for cystitis, vaginal thrush and itching of the vagina or anus.
- Used for a whole host of skin problems – acne, athlete's foot, boils, carbuncles, chicken pox, cuts and wounds, herpes, verrucae and warts.

Special precautions

None. Tea tree is often used neat for first aid purposes.

Remember: always dilute essential oils before using in massage

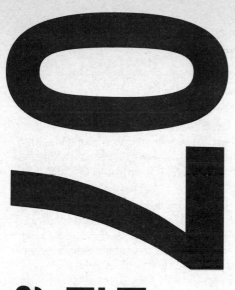

07

massage in pregnancy and childbirth

In this chapter you will learn:
- the importance of massage in pregnancy and labour
- positions for massage
- how to make up essential oil blends for pregnancy, labour and post-natal care.

During the 40 weeks of pregnancy a woman undergoes enormous physical and emotional changes. Massage is an invaluable way to give support to a woman coping with these rapid changes and to prepare her for childbirth. I have treated many patients throughout their pregnancies and they have benefited from massage, enjoying happy and healthy pregnancies and relatively easy deliveries.

Throughout pregnancy chemical drugs (even those taken for common ailments such as headaches or nausea) are contraindicated. They can cross the placenta to the baby and may cause abnormalities in the foetus, particularly during the first few vulnerable months.

Massage, in combination with a healthy diet and exercise, provides a safe, gentle and natural way to relieve the minor discomforts and disorders of pregnancy without the undesirable side-effects of drugs. Of course, if symptoms persist, the mother should always seek the advice of a medical practitioner.

Benefits of massage

A mother-to-be can experience the following benefits from massage:

- a feeling of deep relaxation, extreme tranquillity, optimism and well-being
- a greatly improved sleep pattern
- less fatigue and a boost in energy levels
- back pain is decreased or totally eliminated
- the circulatory and lymphatic systems are stimulated
- fluid retention can be reduced or discouraged
- varicose veins may be avoided or minimized
- aching legs and cramps are relieved
- the frequency of headaches declines
- bowel movements regulate
- stretch marks are prevented
- the perineal area can be prepared for birth
- mood swings and depression induced by hormonal changes are balanced
- breast tenderness is lessened
- posture improves
- the whole body is toned and nourished and the complexion glows

- a strong bond develops between mother-to-be and baby, and both are happy and contented.

Postural changes during pregnancy

Although pregnancy and childbirth are natural processes, pregnancy is one of the most stressful events that can affect a woman's back. The average weight gain is 28 pounds, and approximately 85 per cent of women experience backache during pregnancy. Throughout pregnancy the hormone 'relaxin' is produced to soften and stretch the ligaments in preparation for the birth. As the foetus grows and develops in the uterus, the mother's posture changes dramatically. There is a tendency to overcompensate for the increasing weight of the womb by bending backwards. The lumbar curve increases creating a lordosis (hollow back) in the lumbar spine giving rise to low back ache (see Figure 7.1). The thoracic curve increases making

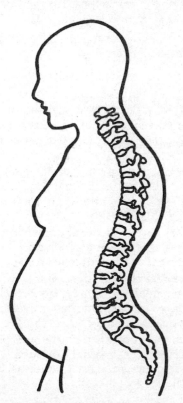

figure 7.1   common posture during pregnancy

a kyphosis (hunch-back) of the upper spine with the head and chin thrown forwards and the shoulders sagging. This results in neck and shoulder tension, and tense, heavy posture is exhausting.

The abdominal muscles are stretched by as much as twice their original length. They usually become weak, lazy and slack, putting strain on the back.

The woman's natural impulse as she gets larger is to stick her stomach out, but she should try to keep her back straight instead of curved. She should be aware of her posture and imagine a cord being pulled upwards from the top of her head, feel her spine lengthening and tuck her tail in to tip her pelvis up and back. Pull back her shoulders, lift her head 'tall' and tuck in her chin. Distribute her body weight evenly onto both feet – if her weight is balanced on one leg this will cause a pelvic tilt and even more strain on her spine. A pregnant woman should not wear high heels since they tip the pelvis forwards, put pressure on the spine and distribute the weight unevenly.

Massage is an excellent way to help the body to cope with these enormous postural changes.

Special considerations

- The massage movements should be soft and gentle and will consist mostly of effleurage. Avoid tapotement. Never apply deep pressure to the abdomen or to the lower back.
- The receiver may need to adopt different positions for massage depending upon the stage of the pregnancy. Except for the early weeks, it is impossible for a mother-to-be to lie prone (face down).
- Take particular care over the abdomen and low back during the first trimester (three months) when working on women who have a history or risk of miscarriage.
- Complications such as high blood pressure, diabetes, anaemia, vaginal bleeding, any fall or accident, or sudden swelling of feet, ankles, fingers or face should always be referred to a qualified medical practitioner.
- Musculo-skeletal problems that are unresponsive to massage are best referred to a qualified osteopath – preferably one who has undergone specialist training in cranial techniques (see 'Useful addresses', p.188).

Check for all the usual contraindications

Positions for massage

Lying on side (semi-prone position)

The pregnant woman lies on her side with her upper knee bent and resting on a pillow. Her head should be well supported on a pillow. Give her as many cushions as she needs for comfort.

Sitting

The pregnant woman should sit astride a chair facing the chair back leaning on pillows or a folded quilt. This position is ideal for both back and neck and shoulder massage.

Lying on back

When the pregnant woman is lying on her back it is essential to put pillows under her knees to relax her abdomen and reduce the curve in her low back.

Remember to cover a pregnant woman with towels exposing only the part of the body that is actually being massaged. The body temperature falls when lying still.

Back

Back pain is particularly common during pregnancy due to the added weight and strain on the muscles and the softening of the ligaments. Backache is one of the most common complaints and a back massage can relieve most of the discomfort. The mother-to-be should adopt either the semi-prone side-lying position or she can sit astride a chair.

Sitting position

1 Start the massage at the bottom of her back, and using the effleurage movements stroke up towards the top of her back, up around her shoulders and glide smoothly down to your starting position with featherlight touch (see Figure 7.2). Repeat these movements until you feel the muscles soften and relax.

2 Place your thumbs in the dimples at the base of her spine and perform the small outward circular friction movements either side of her spine until you reach her neck (see Figure 7.3). Remember to apply only **gentle** pressure in the lumbar area.

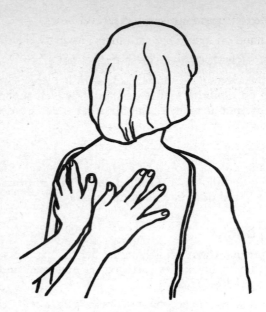

figure 7.2   stroke up the back and over the shoulders

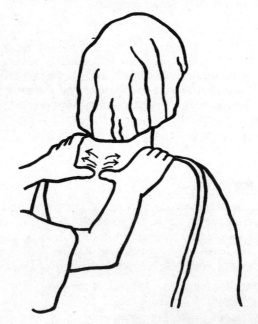

figure 7.3   perform small circular movements either side of the spine

3 Repeat the effleurage movements several times.

4 Rest one hand on one of her shoulders and place the thumb of your other hand between her spine and her shoulder blade. Friction around the border of her shoulder blade.

5 Repeat on the other side of her back changing hands.

6 Squeeze, pick up and wring her shoulder muscles. Work one shoulder at a time for maximum effort.

7 Stand to one side of the pregnant woman. Ask her to flex her head forwards. Place both hands flat down on her neck. Grasp and squeeze her neck muscles **slowly** and **gently** using alternate hands. You may friction her scalp while her head is in this position. Use your fingertips to press firmly into her scalp.

8 *Completion*
Finish with some more effleurage movements, gradually decreasing the pressure.

This massage sequence can also be performed in the semi-prone position with the pregnant woman choosing her most comfortable side to lie on.

Abdomen

Massage of the abdomen is perfectly safe in pregnancy provided that your movements are soft and gentle. Never use deep pressure and percussion movements on the abdomen. Take particular care when working on women who have a history or risk of miscarriage, especially in the first trimester.

The abdomen is the obvious area to massage during pregnancy. It is highly therapeutic for the following reasons:

- It will help to alleviate morning sickness, constipation and diarrhoea, heartburn and indigestion.
- It will help to prevent stretchmarks from appearing.
- The tone of the abdominal muscles will improve, thus allowing the body to cope with the enormous postural changes which occur.
- Massage will encourage the formation of a strong bond between the mother-to-be, the father-to-be and the baby.

Encourage the mother to set aside some time every day to massage her own abdomen and talk to her unborn child. Advise her to massage her perineal area (between the vagina and the anus) particularly towards the end of pregnancy. Use a small amount of carrier oil on the fingertips to massage the perineum. This should reduce the need for stitches.

The best position for abdominal massage is for the pregnant woman to lie on her back with plenty of pillows under her knees to relax the abdomen and to reduce the curve in the lumbar area. Place pillows under the head for comfort.

1 Kneel beside the mother-to-be by her right-hand side and begin to gently effleurage with one hand on top of the other, in a clockwise direction.

2 Continue the effleurage movements but this time use both hands, one hand following the other, working gently and smoothly (see Figure 7.4).

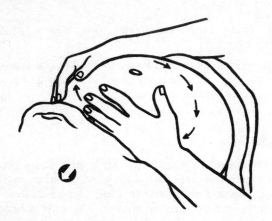

figure 7.4   stroke the abdomen gently in a clockwise direction

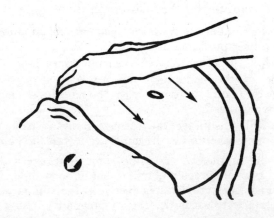

figure 7.5   stroke up the waist

3 Reach over to the opposite side and gently stroke up the waist area. Repeat on the other side (see Figure 7.5).

4 *Completion*
Cover her abdomen with a towel. Place her hands gently over her navel. Leave her to enjoy and establish contact with her baby, who will often respond by kicking or making other movements.

Leg and foot

Leg massage is highly therapeutic and relaxing for the mother-to-be. It improves circulation and can help to relieve and prevent fluid retention, varicose veins, cramps and aches and pains which many women suffer from during pregnancy.

The pregnant woman should adopt a side-lying position. Apply lots of gentle stroking effleurage movements, working from her ankles to her thigh. Always apply pressure on the upwards stroke (see Figure 7.6). If there are varicose veins do not massage **directly** on to the affected veins. You can also perform picking up, rolling and wringing on the thigh. Omit the percussion movements.

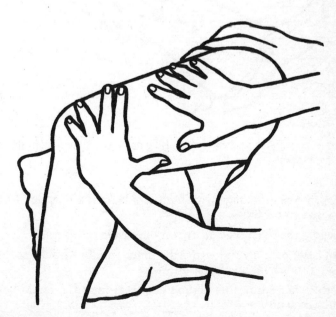

figure 7.6   with the receiver in a side lying position effleurage up the leg

It is also easy to massage the legs and feet while the mother-to-be is lying on her back with plenty of cushions under her knees and under her head. If there is swelling and fluid retention raise her legs slightly.

1 Place one of your hands on the front of her right leg and your other hand on the front of her left leg. Make gentle effleurage movements upwards from her ankles to her thighs on the **front** of her legs, gliding back with no pressure (see Figure 7.7). Repeat these movements several times.

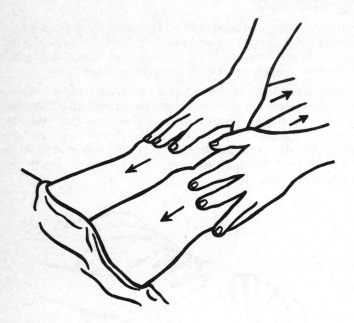

figure 7.7   with the pregnant woman lying on her back the front of the legs may be massaged

2 Repeat the effleurage with both hands on the outside of both her legs several times.

3 Repeat the effleurage gently on the inside of both legs.

4 Squeeze, pick up and wring the inner, middle and outer thigh muscles, working one leg at a time.

5 Stroke her entire foot sliding gently around the ankle bones and back again.

6 Rotate her ankle clockwise and anticlockwise and dorsiflex (pull back) and plantar flex (point) her foot to reduce fluid retention around the vulnerable area.

7 Friction the whole of the sole of her foot starting under her big toe and working outwards. Continue in horizontal rows until the rest of the sole has been completely covered.

8 Repeat steps 5 to 7 on the other foot.

9 *Completion*
Place one hand on each foot and squeeze gently.

Arm, face and breast

Arm

Arm massage is soothing and relaxing and should be performed with the mother-to-be lying on her back propped up on pillows with pillows under her knees. You can follow the complete arm sequence as detailed on pages 47–51 or you can simply effleurage her arms.

Face

Massage on the face is calming and induces feelings of deep relaxation. The mother-to-be can really enjoy being pampered. By the end of the treatment her complexion will feel soft and look glowing. Follow the sequence on pages 58–60 with the pregnant women lying on her back.

Breast

Breasts may seem sore and tender, particularly at the beginning of pregnancy. Self breast massage is recommended for relieving discomfort and preparing the breasts for breast-feeding. Gently cup each breast and effleurage in a circular direction.

Essential oils for pregnancy

Pure essential oils are an invaluable way of enhancing your massage of the mother-to-be. The following recipe makes an ideal general purpose oil for massage during pregnancy.

3 drops of mandarin
3 drops of lavender
2 drops of neroli
} diluted in 20 ml
of carrier oil

You can blend oils to relieve some of the discomforts and problems often experienced in pregnancy, following the recipes listed below.

Backache
Follow the back massage routine already described.

2 drops of Roman chamomile
2 drops of geranium
} diluted in 10 ml
of carrier oil

Constipation
Follow the sequence for abdominal massage.

2 drops of lavender
2 drops of Roman chamomile
} diluted in 10 ml
of carrier oil

Cramp
Follow the routine for leg massage.

1 drop of cypress
1 drop of geranium
2 drops of lavender
} diluted in 10 ml
of carrier oil

Fluid retention
Follow the routine for leg massage.

2 drops of cypress
2 drops of geranium
} diluted in 10 ml
of carrier oil

Heartburn
Follow the abdominal massage sequence.

1 drop of bergamot
1 drop of mandarin
2 drops of sandalwood
} diluted in 10 ml
of carrier oil

Depression/mood swings

Follow the sequence for facial massage.

1 drop of neroli
1 drop of rose   } diluted in 10 ml
2 drops of geranium   of carrier oil

Fatigue

Perform a full massage.

1 drop of geranium
2 drops of lemon   } diluted in 10 ml
1 drop of mandarin   of carrier oil

Anti-stretch marks

Follow the routine for abdominal massage.

2 drops of frankincense
2 drops of lavender
2 drops of mandarin   } diluted in 20 ml
1 drop of neroli   of carrier oil

Varicose veins

Follow the leg massage sequence (gentle movements only).

1 drop of cypress
1 drop of lemon   } diluted in 10 ml
1 drop of geranium   of carrier oil

For more information on the use of essential oils in pregnancy please refer to *Teach Yourself Aromatherapy*.

Massage during labour

During the birth, massage helps to induce feelings of relaxation and calmness. If the massage is performed by the father, it allows him to be part of the experience. It eases pains, especially backache, relaxes the muscles and can help to regulate the contractions and speed up the delivery. Orthodox and complementary pain relief can work hand in hand nowadays – hospital staff respect the mother's preference.

It is difficult to predict what a woman will prefer in labour – what is soothing to one mother would be intensely annoying to another. At some stage of labour she may not even want to be touched. So be flexible and patient. The best areas to massage are the back (especially the lumbar area), shoulders and feet. Use the positions and strokes that I have already described, although a woman will change her position frequently to cope with the pain of the contractions.

Back

The mother-to-be may wish to sit astride a chair or she may find it more comfortable on all fours. Rocking in this position can relieve pain. When she is tired she may wish to lie down on her side in the semi-prone position. Follow the pregnancy back massage routine, which I have already described, with the addition of the following movements to ease the pain.

1 Place your hand flat on the sacrum and apply deep firm pressure. Massage in circular movements using your whole hand. You can also perform these firm, deep, circular pressures over the lumbar area.
2 Press deeply with your thumbs into the centre of each buttock to help to relieve low back pain.
3 Using both hands effleurage from the sacrum out and over the hips and back again.

Abdomen

Effleurage the abdomen in a clockwise direction using featherlight strokes, one hand following the other.

Foot

Firm massage of the feet is relaxing and gives pain relief.

1 Effleurage the feet firmly using both your hands.
2 Press into the soles of the feet with circular movements. Start under the toes and work towards the heel.

You may perform any other movements already described in the previous chapters.

Essential oils for labour

The following recipes will help to ease uterine pain, regulate the contractions, reduce fear and anxiety and boost confidence.

1 drop of rose
1 drop of geranium
2 drops of lavender
} diluted in 10 ml of carrier oil

2 drops of neroli
2 drops of lavender
} diluted in 10 ml of carrier oil

1 drop of jasmine
1 drop of neroli
2 drops of lavender
} diluted in 10 ml of carrier oil

Post-natal massage

In many cultures massage is an essential part of post-natal care. In parts of the East, a woman is massaged every day for at least a month after giving birth. After each massage her abdomen is bound with long strips of cloth.

Massage after delivery gives the following benefits:

- the abdominal muscles are encouraged to contract to their normal size and regain their tone
- involution is aided (the time taken for the womb to return to its normal size)
- massage helps to combat the effects of tension and tiredness
- the woman feels nurtured and is restored emotionally at a time when the sudden change of hormone levels can lead to post-natal depression.

Special considerations

- Do not massage scar area on the abdomen after a Caesarean section (but massage all other areas).
- In the first few days following any birth it is often possible to give only gentle effleurage of the abdomen.

Massage movements

1 Squeeze, roll and wring the waist, hips and thighs to break up the fatty tissue, which has accumulated during pregnancy.

2 Perform effleurage and gentle wringing on the abdomen to induce muscle tone and to reduce any stretch marks.

All areas of the body will benefit from massage in the post-natal period. Follow sequences in Chapter 04 paying attention to the abdomen.

Essential oils for post-natal care

Keep using the anti-stretch mark oil described above while the body is returning to normal. The mother can still get stretch marks after the birth as her weight decreases.

Post-natal blues

| 1 drop of rose
1 drop of bergamot
1 drop of geranium | or | 1 drop of jasmine
1 drop of neroli
1 drop of mandarin | diluted in
10 ml of
carrier oil |

Post-natal energizer

| 1 drop of rosemary
1 drop of lemon
1 drop of frankincense | diluted in
10 ml of
carrier oil |

Healing the perineum

| 2 drops of lavender
1 drop of Roman chamomile | diluted in 10 ml
of carrier oil |

Breast massage

Wash any oil off the nipple before breastfeeding.

| 2 drops of neroli
2 drops of geranium | diluted in 10 ml
of carrier oil |

For further information on the use of aromatherapy in pregnancy, childbirth and after delivery please refer to *Teach Yourself Aromatherapy*.

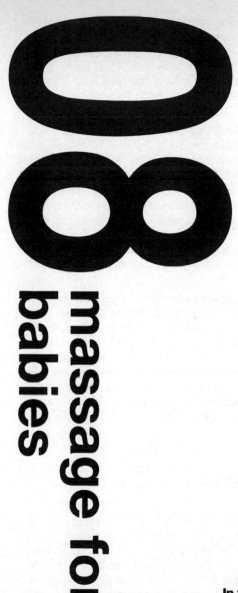

08

massage for babies

In this chapter you will learn:
- the benefits of baby massage
- how to perform a complete baby massage
- how to make up essential oil blends for babies and children.

Touch is the first sense developed by the embryo as it is rocked and massaged in the womb, surrounded by the amniotic fluid. As the baby is gradually pushed down the birth canal he or she is receiving a stimulating massage to prepare him or her to adapt to the new environment. After babies have made their difficult journey into the world they need the constant reassurance of a loving touch.

Massage has been practised for centuries in many cultures, and nowadays in parts of India, Pakistan, some African countries and the West Indies, massage is part of a baby's daily life. Babies are massaged almost as soon as they are born, often initially by their grandmothers. The mother takes over the daily ritual when she feels fit. The practice of massage continues throughout life, and children and adults are frequently massaged. Massage creates a strong and loving link between mother, father and baby. The London obstetrician Yehudi Gordon states that 'massage helps parents communicate with their baby, thereby strengthening the bonding process'.

Touch is particularly important for premature babies and those in special care if bonding is to be established. Babies who are born by Caesarean section and thus are not massaged through the birth canal also require a great deal of touch. Fast-birth babies who can be traumatized and shocked by the speed of the delivery also need massage. It assists in the physiological and emotional development of the child. Evidence suggests that babies who receive regular massage are subject to far fewer health problems. They also feed and sleep much better than those who receive no massage.

Benefits of massage

Digestive system

Both digestion and elimination is improved. Many mothers report that massage helps their babies to suckle better, leading to an improved feeding pattern. Babies suffer from far less colic, constipation and diarrhoea. In my practice I see an increasing number of babies and children who have constipation problems. I am shocked that they are prescribed medications which can become addictive at such a young age, when all that is necessary is a daily abdominal massage and sometimes a change of diet.

Nervous system

It is remarkable how babies can be calmed and even lulled to sleep after a short massage treatment. Irritability, frustration and temper tantrums are reduced, resulting in much easier nights for the parents. Massage is as beneficial for the parents' state of mind as it is for the baby – parents become much less agitated and more able to cope with all the pressures and worries of a new baby. Calmness and tranquillity can be restored.

Immune system

Babies who are massaged are far more resistant to infections and experience far fewer health problems. I have two children, one of 11 years and one of 13 years, and they have never required any antibiotics or drugs of any description – not even 'Calpol'!

Respiratory system

Some babies always seem to be full of mucus. Massage will result in fewer coughs, colds, nasal problems and ear infections.

Musculo-skeletal system

Baby massage will encourage the joints and muscles to become flexible and supple and enables the baby to co-ordinate its muscular movements.

Skin

The texture, tone and condition of the baby's skin will improve with regular massage. The blood circulation is activated and any waste products are rapidly removed from the system. The baby's skin will look healthy and glowing after treatment.

Emotions

Babies and children who are massaged appear to experience fewer emotional or psychological problems later in life. They are more confident, independent and secure, and are more well-balanced.

According to Stuart Korth, founder of the Osteopathic Centre for Children, nine out of ten children suffer some trauma in the birth process. I strongly agree that every child should be checked at birth to reduce and normalize imbalances and restore and maintain health.

The cranial approach to osteopathy is a gentle, safe and non-invasive form of treatment. The osteopath's highly developed sense of touch is used to identify and correct disturbances and limitations both within the bones of the skull and throughout the body. The medical profession is becoming increasingly aware of the benefits of osteopathy in the cranial field. Referrals are regularly received from paediatricians, midwives, health visitors and other health care professionals. A consultation with an osteopath who has received further training in paediatrics and is experienced in this field is vital. I recommend that you take your baby or child to the Osteopathic Centre for Children, where I received superb training (see 'Useful addresses', p.188).

Special considerations

- Ensure that the room is extremely warm. The baby will be naked for the massage and babies lose heat rapidly and feel the cold much more quickly than adults.
- Always be responsive to the mood of your baby and massage only when the time is right. Don't attempt to massage a baby who is hungry, restless, irritable or overtired. You can perform the massage at any time of the day – about half an hour or so after a feed or after bathtime is best. If the baby is not enjoying the massage then stop immediately and try again later.
- Ensure that you are also in the right mood. If you are tired, irritable, depressed or in a hurry these feeling will be communicated to the baby. Babies are highly intuitive.
- Babies have a short attention span and tire easily. Ten minutes will probably be sufficient.
- Ensure that everything you will need is close at hand before you begin – oil, towels, blankets, clean nappy, tissues and clothes.
- Check that your nails are short and remove any jewellery prior to a massage.
- It is a good idea to start the massage on the front of the baby's body to establish eye contact, trust and security.
- Talk to the baby reassuringly throughout the massage to make the experience as enjoyable as possible.
- If the navel is still healing, take care not to touch it.
- Lay a towel on the floor in case of accidents. A baby will usually empty its bladder during the massage.
- Make sure that your hands are warm before massaging the baby. An abrupt change in temperature may induce crying.
- Warm the oil to hand temperature by putting the bottle in a bowl containing hot water for a few minutes.

Positions for massage

1 When massaging a young baby sit on the floor with your legs together stretched out in front of you. You may bring your knees up slightly by placing a pillow underneath them so that the baby is resting on your thighs **OR**

2 Place a thick duvet on the floor and cover it with a warm, soft towel.

Baby massage oil

A light vegetable oil easily absorbed by the skin such as sweet almond oil is perfect for your massage. Remember to use only cold pressed, unrefined vegetable oils (see pages 12–14). Mineral oils are not suitable as they tend to clog pores and do not penetrate easily.

The following aromatic recipe may be used as a general massage oil. I suggest that you make up a 50 ml bottle.

1 drop of Roman chamomile
1 drop of lavender   } diluted in 50 ml
1 drop of neroli   of carrier oil
1 drop of rose

Do not be tempted to use more drops of essential oils – babies and young children require a low amount of essential oils. Too much is harmful.

Suggested routine

There is no definitive sequence for massaging babies, and you will develop your own routine. Listen to your intuition and be adaptable. Perform each movement several times.

Legs and front of body

A baby is fascinated by its toes and will love to watch you as you massage. Lay the baby on its back.

1 Pour some oil on to your hands and rub it gently into the baby's leg. Hold the foot and effleurage the leg from ankle to thigh (see Figure 8.1) Allow your hands to glide gently down with no pressure. Repeat this effleurage several times.

2 Gently twist your hands in a corkscrew action, beginning at the ankle and working up the thigh (see Figure 8.2).

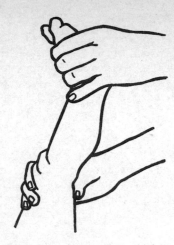

figure 8.1 effleurage baby's leg from ankle to thigh

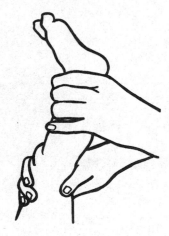

figure 8.2 work up baby's leg using a twisting action

3 Hold the foot and gently massage the sole of the foot with your thumb using circular movements (see Figure 8.3).

4 Slowly and gently circumduct the foot clockwise and then anticlockwise.

5 Support the foot with one hand. Squeeze each toe between the index finger and the thumb.

6 Bend and stretch the knee slowly (see Figure 8.4).

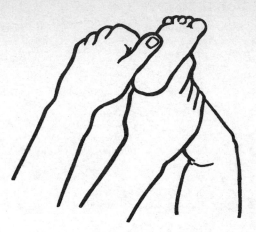

figure 8.3   use gentle circular movements on the sole of baby's foot

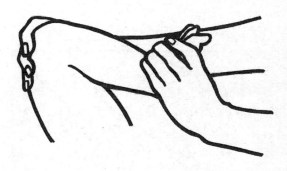

figure 8.4   gently bend and stretch the knee

7 *Completion*
Effleurage the entire leg again, gradually decreasing the pressure.

Repeat these movements on the other leg

Chest and abdomen

1 With both hands slowly and gently effleurage up the front of the body. Allow the hands to glide back (see Figure 8.5).

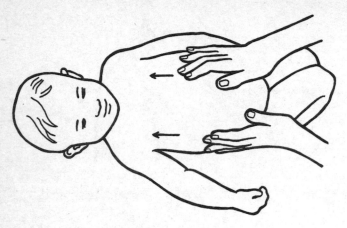

figure 8.5 gently stroke up the front of the baby

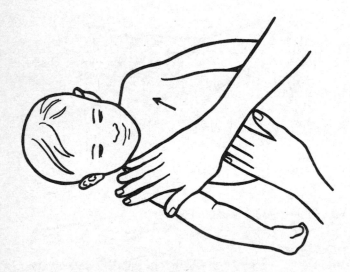

figure 8.6 effleurage baby using a criss-cross action

2 Crossing effleurage

Place both hands at the bottom of the trunk. Effleurage your right hand up towards the **left** shoulder. The moment the **right** hand reaches the opposite shoulder, effleurage your **left** hand towards the right shoulder (see Figure 8.6). Repeat these movements with a slow steady rhythm.

3 Place both your hands on the baby's chest and lightly stroke outwards across the top of the chest (see Figure 8.7).

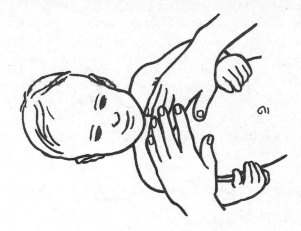

figure 8.7   gently stroke across baby's chest

4 Using flat fingers circle all over the chest area.

5 Rest both hands on the abdomen, one on top of the other and with featherlight touch move in a clockwise direction (see Figure 8.8). These movements are excellent for colic, constipation and other digestive upsets.

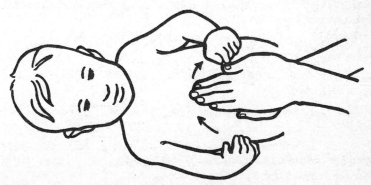

figure 8.8   stroke baby's abdomen in a circular direction

6 *Completion*
Repeat the effleurage with both hands gliding up the front of the body towards the shoulders and back again.

Arms and hands

The baby should either continue to lie on his or her back or if old enough may sit up.

1 Hold the baby's hand and gently and slowly effleurage from the fingers to the shoulder (see Figure 8.9). Glide down again.

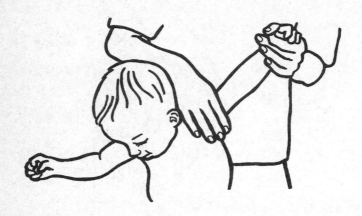

figure 8.9 effleurage up baby's arm

2 Gently twist your hands in a corkscrew motion progressing from the wrist up to the shoulder (see Figure 8.10).

3 Open the baby's hand. Support the back of the hand, and using your fingers gently effleurage over the palm using circular movements.

4 Massage each finger in turn by gently unfolding them one after the other.

5 Slowly and gently circumduct the wrist clockwise and anticlockwise.

6 Flex and extend the baby's elbow gently and slowly.

7 *Completion*
Hold the baby's hand and repeat the effleurage from the fingers to the shoulders. Finish by gently holding the baby's hand between your cupped palms.

Repeat these movements on the other arm

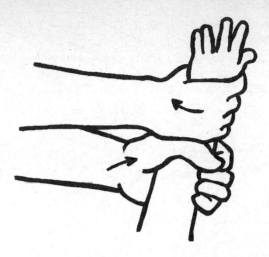

figure 8.10 use a corkscrew action working from waist to shoulder

Face

The facial massage should be performed with a light touch. This is one of the most rewarding areas to treat. You can enjoy total eye contact with the baby. Always take care not to apply oil near the baby's eyes.

1 Stroke gently down the sides of the baby's face from the top to the chin (see Figure 8.11).

2 Using the tips of your fingers stroke the baby's forehead from the middle out towards the hairline.

3 With gentle thumb pressure start at the nose and the cheeks. Repeat to cover the entire cheek area (see Figure 8.12).

4 Place your thumb under the lower lip and stroke outwards across the chin.

5 With your index fingers, make gentle circles around the eye area and also around the mouth.

6 *Completion*
To connect the front of the baby's body stroke your hands from the top of the head, down the torso and down the legs.

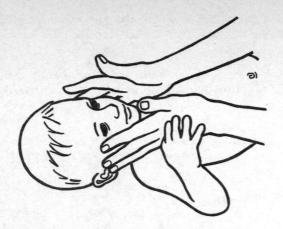

figure 8.11   stroke gently down the sides of baby's face

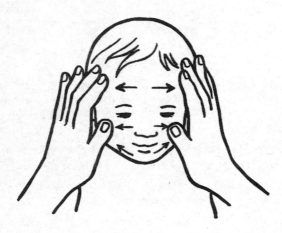

figure 8.12   stroke outwards across the face

Back of the body

Turn baby over and lay it on it's tummy. The baby can either lie on the duvet on the floor or sideways across your thighs rather than along them.

1 Effleurage from the buttocks up the back and over the shoulders returning to your starting position with absolutely no pressure (see Figure 8.13).

2 Place both hands flat down on the buttocks and perform circular stroking movements over each buttock.

3 Gently squeeze the buttocks.

4 To connect the back of the body and conclude the massage glide both hands from baby's head down the back towards the feet.

5 *Completion*
Bring the baby close to you and finish with a cuddle. After being massaged babies often fall into a contented and deeply relaxed sleep.

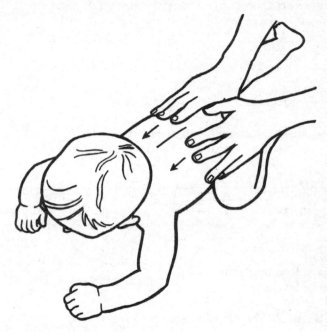

figure 8.13   stroke gently up baby's back

Essential oils for baby

The baby massage oil that I described on page 105 will be perfect for your massage. However, the following blends may be helpful if problems do occur.

Naturally, if you are at all concerned about your baby's health you should seek medical advice immediately. I have included dosages for children, who are just as easy to massage as babies.

Children of all ages will thoroughly enjoy and respond extremely well to regular massage. Be creative with your movements and adapt the routines already given depending on the needs of your child.

Suitable dilutions are as follows:

Babies (0–2 months)	1 drop per 15 ml carrier oil
Babies (2–12 months)	1 drop per 10 ml carrier oil
Small children (up to 5 years)	2 drops per 10 ml carrier oil
Juniors (5 to 12 years)	2–3 drops per 10 ml carrier oil

Remember **never** to use commercial baby oil as a carrier. It is a mineral oil and will not penetrate the skin.

Colic
1 drop of Roman chamomile diluted in 15 ml carrier oil

Massage gently on to baby's tummy, back and feet in a clockwise direction.

Coughs/colds/respiratory problems
1 drop of lavender/frankincense diluted in 20 ml carrier oil

Nappy rash
3 drops of Roman chamomile } in a 60 g jar of pure organic
2 drops of lavender } skin cream or zinc and castor oil cream

Teething
1 drop of Roman chamomile } diluted in 15 ml carrier oil
1 drop of lavender }

Massage gently into the cheeks.

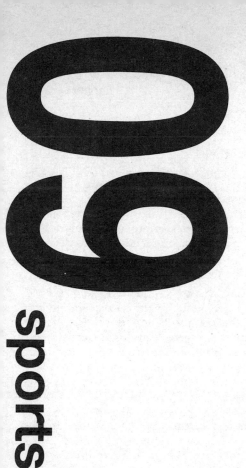

09

sports injuries

In this chapter you will learn:
- the importance of pre-event and post-event massage
- self-help for acute injuries
- how to deal with the most common sports injuries.

If we could give every individual the right amount of nourishment and exercise, not too little and not too much, we would have found the safest way to health.

Hippocrates

The importance of exercise

In this stressful age we should strive for physical fitness. Exercise and sport, if performed correctly and sensibly, will make you feel lighter in both mind and body and well equipped to cope with all the pressures of everyday life. Exercise is essential for good health. The benefits of exercise are numerous – the function of the heart and lungs improves, circulation is stimulated, muscles and joints become more supple and flexible, digestive problems subside and the immune system is boosted allowing the body to become more resistant to disease.

There has been a tremendous increase in the numbers of people participating in sport and attending health clubs and gyms. Unfortunately this has resulted in an upsurge in the number of sports injuries. These injuries are often due to unaccustomed exercise, for instance, when an individual with a sedentary job engages in a vigorous high-impact aerobics class after 15 years of almost total inactivity – not a good idea! It is essential to begin gradually when embarking upon an exercise régime, doing a little at each session, **progressively** increasing the amount that you do. Little and often is the golden rule. If you are unused to exercise you should seek professional advice as to what kind of exercise or sport would be suitable for you.

You should take exercise on a regular basis and this, of course, should go hand in hand with a healthy diet. Avoid 'junk' food as much as possible and eat a healthy, balanced diet with lots of fresh fruit and vegetables. Follow the wise words of Hippocrates.

Do not exercise or take part in sport either directly after a heavy meal or on a completely empty stomach. A light snack about an hour or two beforehand will suffice. In order to avoid cramp and dehydration be aware of your fluid intake. Always carry a bottle of water with you when you exercise.

Never play sport when you are feeling unwell or generally below par. A virus or infection will invariably worsen after exercise and in extreme cases may result in death.

Before any sporting activity you must prepare yourself properly. Always warm up and stretch your body gently, and at the end of the session warm down thoroughly.

The benefits of massage

When injury does strike, massage is a highly effective treatment for the majority of complaints and is an excellent aid to recuperation.

- Massage increases blood flow both into and out of the affected areas, thus speeding up the healing process considerably.
- Massage stimulates the elimination of accumulated metabolic waste. As a result of exercise waste products such as lactic acid and urea, which are released into and build up in the muscles, may crystallize inducing cramps, stiffness, pain and soreness. These may be dispelled easily by soft tissue work after exercise.
- Massage provides pain relief by stretching the soft tissues and releasing endorphins.
- Elasticity and pliability of the tissues will improve. It will help prevent formation of adhesions or scar tissue. Old scar tissue and adhesions in muscles, tendons and ligaments, which have built up as a result of previous traumas, can be broken down effectively.
- Massage should be seen as a preventive medicine. It is excellent for the avoidance of overuse injuries and should be employed on a regular basis to relieve any minor aches or pains, which could eventually lead to trauma. Many sportsmen and sportswomen have massage therapy to reduce nervous tension and to relax the mind before an important event.

Pre-event massage

The primary function of pre-event massage is to invigorate rather than relax. Muscles need to be loosened and warmed and prepared for work before an event. This will increase performance, stamina and agility and minimize the likelihood of muscle strains occurring during the event. In a pre-event massage, the massage movements will be vigorous and stimulating.

Pre-event essential oils

2 drops of black pepper ⎫
2 drops of ginger   ⎬ or
2 drops of rosemary   ⎭

1 drop of eucalyptus ⎫ diluted in
2 drops of lemon   ⎪ 20 ml
1 drop of peppermint ⎬ of
2 drops of rosemary ⎭ carrier oil

Post-event massage

The main objective of post-event massage is to allow the muscles to recover from fatigue. The massage aims to eliminate waste products such as lactic acid and other deposits from the tissues. Top sportsmen and women can accelerate their recovery time from three days to just one day. In a post-event massage, the movements will be slow and firm to promote the cleansing action.

Post-event essential oils

2 drops of Roman chamomile ⎫
1 drop of cypress   ⎪
2 drops of frankincense   ⎬ or
                           ⎪
1 drop of juniper   ⎭

1 drop of frankincense ⎫ diluted
2 drops of juniper   ⎪ in
2 drops of marjoram   ⎬ 20 ml
                       ⎪ of
1 drop of lavender   ⎭ carrier oil

Treatment

You must **never** diagnose. All injuries should be examined and diagnosed by a qualified medical practitioner before starting treatment. Certain injuries require investigation by X-ray and blood tests. If you ignore an injury you could suffer serious long-term damage. However, after the initial diagnosis self-help massage can be beneficial, but you should **never** attempt to 'work through' the pain as this will damage the injured tissues even further.

When not to massage

- Do not massage open wounds. Begin treatment only when the scar has started to form (a week or so, depending on the severity of the injury). After this you can massage gently around the scar but not directly on to it until the scar has completely healed, which could take a few months.
- Do not massage fractures. Start treatment only after the cast has been removed.

- Do not massage where an acute inflammatory condition is present, indicated by swelling, heat, redness and stiffness. Acute inflammation will be present in diseases such as rheumatoid arthritis and gout. Any condition with 'itis' on the end is an inflammatory condition (e.g. bursitis).

- Do not massage in cases of thrombo-phlebitis. Treatment could cause the thrombus (clot) to move and could be fatal. If there is a possibility of thrombosis, seek medical advice.

- Do not massage during infectious conditions. The infection could be transmitted to other parts of the body and also to the therapist. Infectious conditions include measles, chicken pox, herpes, scabies, impetigo, warts, verrucae, ringworm and athlete's foot.

- Do not massage over unidentified lumps and bumps. If treatment is applied to malignant tumours, they could spread.

- Do not apply massage until at least 48 hours after an injury has occurred.

Acute injuries

Bleeding, swelling, pain and tenderness are all signs of a sudden injury. Treatment is usually:

R = Rest
I = Ice
C = Compression
E = Elevation

RICE treatment minimizes bleeding and swelling and reduces pain, and it should help to prevent the formation of chronic adhesions and scar tissue.

Rest

Immobilizing the injured part reduces the pain and swelling and prevents further injury to the soft tissues. Splints and bandages are often used to support the affected area. A sling is useful for an injured arm. In severe cases a cast will be applied.

Ice

Ice gives local pain relief, reduces bleeding (as it slows down the blood circulation and contracts the blood vessels) and prevents further swelling.

Cold treatments are applied locally to the injured area, either an ice pack or a wet towel containing ice cubes or a packet of frozen food. Ice placed directly on to the skin could cause an ice-burn. Use cold therapy every four hours after an injury. The ice pack should be removed when the skin has turned pink or if it becomes uncomfortable.

Never apply heat immediately after an acute injury as it will increase swelling and internal bleeding, causing severe pain and delaying the healing process. Heat may be recommended a few days after the injury to relieve muscle tension.

Aromatherapy compresses

Hot and cold aromatherapy compresses are invaluable in the treatment of sports injuries. For acute pain or hot swellings use a cold compress. Post-acute or chronic injuries require hot compresses or a combination of hot and cold.

To make a compress mix six drops of pure essential oil into a small bowl of water. Soak any piece of absorbent material such as a flannel, piece of sheeting or towelling in the solution to absorb as much as possible. Gently squeeze the compress and apply it to the injured part. Wrap clingfilm around it to stop it from dripping everywhere and leave it for about two hours or even overnight.

Compression

A compression bandage may prevent further swelling and reduce bleeding. A hard pad is applied to the site of the injury and then bound firmly but not too tightly with an elastic bandage.

Elevation

Elevation of the injured part will reduce the blood flow and minimise the swelling considerably. If the limb is not raised then gravity will increase the swelling and irritation. Support a swollen leg at an angle of more than 45° using a few cushions under the leg. If the lower arm is swollen use a sling to help fluid flow. If the upper part of the arm is swollen, the patient should raise the arm over his or her head at frequent intervals.

Further treatment

Two to three days after an acute injury massage is usually beneficial but it should take the form of gentle superficial movements. Stop the massage immediately if there is pain.

Heat treatment is often recommended for post-acute injuries, or a combination of hot and cold treatment. Remember to use only cold therapy immediately after an injury, as heat will increase swelling. Wait at least 48 hours after an acute injury before starting heat treatment.

When all the redness has disappeared, heat is beneficial for relieving muscle tension and increasing circulation. You can buy specially made hot-and-cold packs or you may use a packet of frozen foods and a hot-water bottle. Apply heat for one minute followed by cold for one minute and repeat this procedure three or four times. Protect the skin with a towel to avoid burns and soreness.

Contrast baths are also recommended. Prepare two buckets/bowls of water – one iced and the other as hot as the patient is able to tolerate. Dip the injured part into one bucket for a few seconds and then take it out and immerse it in the other bucket. Repeat this procedure for about ten minutes. It will increase the blood and lymph flow, reduce pain and accelerate the healing process considerably.

A–Z of sports injuries

Achilles tendinitis

Inflammation of the tendon causes pain, and limits movement. Achilles tendinitis may be caused by running on hard surfaces for long periods.

Treatment

In the acute phase apply ice packs followed by hot and cold therapy. Aromatherapy compresses using Roman chamomile reduce inflammation. Essential oil of peppermint is marvellous for reducing pain.

Effleurage along the sides of the Achilles tendon, with the receiver's lower leg raised to encourage drainage and reduce swelling. Apply friction massage to break down adhesions and to improve the circulation.

Tendinitis essential oils

1 drop of frankincense   } diluted in 10 ml
1 drop of peppermint   } of carrier oil

Runners who suffer from Achilles tendinitis should check their shoes – high heel tabs can cause Achilles tendinitis and the heel tab may need to be cut away.

Athlete's foot (*tinea pedis*)

The warm, damp conditions inside training shoes and in changing rooms are ideal for the development of the fungal infection known as 'athlete's foot'. The fungus makes the skin between the toes moist, cracked and whitish in appearance. The skin will itch and can be painful if the cracks deepen. There may also be an offensive smell. The fungus is infectious and is easily spread via floors on which people walk barefoot.

Treatment

This fungal infection can be persistent and difficult to eradicate with orthodox medicine. The essential oils, lavender, myrrh and tea tree are all fungicidal and are excellent for healing athlete's foot.

Athlete's foot essential oils

Bathe the feel daily in a bowl of water to which you have added:

2 drops of lavender
2 drops of myrrh   or   1 drop of lavender
2 drops of tea tree   2 drops of tea tree

You may also use neat lavender or tea tree. Use a cotton bud to apply it between the toes and around the nails where the fungus can multiply. A massage oil can also be rubbed into the feet as a preventive measure:

1 drop of lavender   diluted in
1 drop of lemon   10 ml of
1 drop of tea tree   carrier oil

To prevent a reoccurrence wash the feet regularly and thoroughly dry them afterwards. Wear socks made of natural materials such as wool or cotton and change them frequently. Sufferers should avoid going barefoot in changing rooms and swimming pools and should not allow anyone else to use their towels, shoes or socks.

Blisters

Blisters are caused by friction due to unaccustomed or prolonged rubbing – for example by shoes or by the handle of a tennis or squash racket, cricket bat and so on. Blisters are more likely to occur in hot weather as the hands and feet may swell creating a different grip or more compression in the shoes. Blisters may seem a trivial injury, but they can result in long breaks from training, particularly if an infection develops.

Treatment

Ensure that your footwear fits properly and is properly worn in. Check that your racket is the correct size. Take care of your feet with regular aromatherapy footbaths – six drops of pure essential oil to a bowl of water. Benzoin, myrrh, lavender and tea tree are particularly beneficial.

For a minor blister apply a few drops of neat pure essential oil of tea tree or lavender to the area and protect it from further friction with a gauze dressing held in place with plaster strips so that the air can get in.

If the blister is large, puncture it by making two small holes at the end of it with a **sterilized** needle and gently squeeze out the fluid. Then protect the area with a plaster.

Keep blisters scrupulously clean. Leave shoes or socks off for as much time as possible to encourage healing.

Blister essential oil

Dab blisters with a strong solution of tea tree – six drops to an egg-cup full of water.

Bruises

Treatment

As soon as possible after the bruising has occurred wrap some ice cubes in a towel and place this on the affected area. Alternately use an ice-cold compress.

2 drops of geranium 2 drops of lavender 2 drops of rosemary }	diluted in a small bowl of cold water and applied as a compress

The homoeopathic remedy Arnica is also extremely effective.

As the bruise develops and begins to turn green or yellow, massage the affected area to help disperse the bruise. Massage will increase the local circulation and encourage the blood which was released into the surrounding tissues to drain way.

Bruises essential oils

1 drop of black pepper 1 drop of geranium 1 drop of lavender 1 drop of rosemary }	diluted in 10 ml of carrier oil

Cuts and wounds

Cuts and wounds are extremely common in contact sports, athletics and cycling. Wash all skin wounds thoroughly as even a minor cut carries a risk of infection. Essential oils are antiseptic and therefore ideal for cleansing and treating wounds. They also help to stop bleeding, promote healing and have pain relieving properties too.

Treatment

Stop the bleeding
If the wound is severe, basic first aid is required. Raise the injured part and then apply direct pressure to the wound. Place a pressure bandage over the injured area and consult a doctor.

If the wound is less serious, diluted essential oil of lemon speeds up the coagulation of blood and stops the flow of blood. It is also antiseptic. Freshly squeezed lemon juice is just as effective if the essential oil is unavailable. Soak a pad of gauze in the diluted lemon – three drops to 10 ml of water – and press it firmly against the wound. Essential oil of geranium also stops bleeding.

Nosebleeds are common in contact sports such as football, rugby, ice-hockey and boxing. To control a nosebleed sit the patient down with head forwards and use your thumb and index finger to pinch the nostrils together, maintaining the pressure for about ten minutes until the bleeding has stopped. Do **not** tip the head backwards as blood may run down the back of the throat. The casualty should breathe through his or her mouth. Inhale essential oil of lemon or freshly squeezed lemon juice. Once the bleeding is under control, gently clean the nose and mouth area. The casualty should **not** blow the nose or the clot could be disturbed.

Clean and dress the wound
It is vital to remove all dirt otherwise bacteria will begin to multiply, invading the tissues and resulting in infection. Bathe the area thoroughly in the following solution:

> 5 drops of lavender } diluted in 1 pint
> 5 drops of tea tree } of warm water

After the wound has been cleansed thoroughly, apply a drop of neat lavender or neat tea tree. It may sting slightly but it is not as uncomfortable as disinfectant.

If the cut is superficial, allow the damaged skin to heal in the fresh air to accelerate the healing process. Otherwise put three drops of lavender or tea tree on a piece of gauze or on a plaster and place it over the cut.

If in any doubt as to the severity of the wound, refer to a qualified medical practitioner.

Fractures

A fracture is a **serious** injury to the skeleton and to the surrounding tissues – tendons, ligaments, muscles, nerves, blood vessels and skin – indicated by:

- deformity and abnormal mobility of the injured bone
- extreme tenderness around the site of the injury
- swelling and bruising caused by damage to the soft tissues and blood vessels.

Treatment

If you suspect a fracture, massage is absolutely forbidden. You could do considerable damage by massaging over the site of even the smallest break. For example, a splinter of bone could lacerate an artery, nerve or a vein. A qualified remedial masseur would have the knowledge to administer treatment almost immediately, but you should **not** attempt any treatment until the bone is mended. Cover the open injury with a clean bandage, immobilize the limb and raise it. Take the casualty to the hospital immediately, where a plaster cast will be applied.

Once the cast has been removed, with the doctor's permission, you can begin gentle effleurage of the limb in the direction of the venous flow. Massage treatment can relieve muscular spasm and pain and help to restore muscle tone.

Golfer's elbow

This condition is also known as 'thrower's elbow' or medial epicondylitis and is similar to 'tennis elbow' except the symptoms are located on the medial (inner) side of the elbow. The problem arises from the medial epicondyle where the flexor muscles of the forearm attach. The sufferer feels pain on the medial aspect of the elbow with referred pain into the wrist and fingers and even up into the shoulder.

Golfer's elbow is much less common than tennis elbow. It is most prevalent in 'throwing' sports such as javelin, cricket, baseball and racket sports. A right-handed golf player may be unfortunate enough to suffer from tennis elbow in the leading left elbow and golfer's elbow in the following right elbow.

If you do play golf then try not to spend more than one hour at a driving range and rest frequently. Try to have regular massage and apply self-massage before and after playing, at the first sign of tenderness. Strengthen your forearm muscles with regular exercise.

Treatment

Golfer's elbow requires rest and, if the pain is intense, hot and cold therapy – cold therapy only in the acute stages and cold and hot therapy after a couple of days. Compression bandaging and elevation are not necessary.

Massage is invaluable in the treatment of this condition. Effleurage the whole arm and pay particular attention to the forearm. Hold the forearm up from the waist with the arm in an outwardly rotated position so that you can treat the flexor muscles. Apply deep effleurage and friction to this area. Where there is pain in the wrist and fingers massage the hand and wrist.

Golfer's elbow essential oils

1 drop of Roman chamomile } diluted in 10 ml
1 drop of lavender   of carrier oil
1 drop of peppermint

Shin splints

This condition, otherwise known as medial tibial stress syndrome, is particularly common in long distance runners who subject themselves to intensive training sessions on hard tracks or roads. The pain is felt along the medial side of the tibia (shin) particularly in the lower half of the tibia. There is some swelling and the medial border of the tibia is tender.

Treatment

'Shin splints' can develop suddenly after acute overuse or impact trauma. Administer treatment immediately to avoid a chronic condition. Stop training straight away and have complete rest. Do not resume training until there is no more tenderness. Apply ice packs to reduce the inflammation and pain. Aromatherapy cold compresses with six drops of Roman chamomile will also relieve the inflammation. After 48 hours apply alternating hot and cold compresses using three drops of peppermint and three drops of lavender.

After the inflammation has subsided massage the whole of the lower leg and foot. Pain from shin splints is triggered when the toes or ankle joint are bent downwards. Effleurage the entire lower leg and apply friction along the medial border of the tibia to help to break down adhesions. Perform picking up, rolling and wringing movements over the gastrocnemius and soleus muscles at the back of the calf. Effleurage the foot and mobilize the ankle. There will be an excellent response to the treatment if massage is administered on a daily basis.

If the condition persists consult a qualified medical practitioner who may want to take an X-ray. There may be a stress fracture.

To avoid medial tibial stress syndrome choose well fitting running shoes to suit the surface. The muscles should be thoroughly warmed up and stretched before a run and the legs should be massaged regularly on a weekly basis.

Shin splints essential oils

1 drop of Roman chamomile
1 drop of lavender
1 drop of peppermint
} diluted in 10 ml of carrier oil

Sprains

A sprain is a **joint** injury that occurs when a joint is wrenched and forced beyond its natural range of motion. A sprain affects the soft tissues around the joint – ligaments, muscles, tendons and so on. Symptoms include pain, swelling and loss of movement. The most commonly affected areas are the ankles and wrists. Most sportsmen and women will suffer at some time from a sprained ankle – runners, tennis and squash players, football and rugby players are particularly susceptible. Awkward twists, sudden impacts and falls are common causes.

Treatment

Apply ice packs or cold compresses immediately until the acute stage is over. Essential oils of lavender and chamomile are excellent in compresses for giving pain relief and reducing inflammation.

Raise the limb and rest it as much as possible. Strapping is often necessary to provide support. Massage can be applied daily after the tenderness has subsided.

Ankle sprain

After the acute phase effleurage first from knee to thigh and then from ankle to knee to help disperse the swelling. As the injury heals gently knead and friction, gradually increasing the pressure. Deep friction applied after five or six days helps to prevent the formation of scar tissue and adhesions. When the pain has subsided gently mobilize the ankle. Dorsiflex, plantar flex and circumduct the ankle to help to restore full movement.

Sprains essential oils

2 drops of Roman chamomile } diluted in 10 ml
2 drops of peppermint diluted in 10 ml of carrier oil

Strains

Muscle injuries are among the most common conditions in sports medicine and account for up to a third of all sporting injuries. A strain occurs when a muscle is abnormally stretched. Symptoms include pain, stiffness, swelling and loss of full power. Strains in the hamstring muscles are common in sports involving rapid flexion of the knee such as running, jumping, football and racket sports. Strains in the quadriceps muscles are frequent in sports such as sprinting and jumping and are usually sustained at the 'take off'. The gastrocnemius muscle is often strained in sports involving running on hard surfaces such as squash, badminton and tennis. Abdominal muscle strains are sustained in sports such as gymnastics, weightlifting, skating and pole vaulting where extension of the back and hip is required.

Treatment

Muscle strains **must** be rested. Massage movements must **not** be applied until the acute stage has passed. Apply cold therapy in the initial stages followed by hot and cold therapy. You may also apply aromatherapy compresses.

When the acute stage has passed after two to three days then perform gentle effleurage. The aim is to improve circulation, remove scar tissue and strengthen the muscle. As the muscle strain heals, kneading and friction are effective treatments.

Strains essential oils

The following essential oils will provide pain relief, stimulate blood and lymph flow, reduce inflammation and encourage muscle tone and function.

1 drop of rosemary ⎫
1 drop of lavender ⎬ diluted in 10 ml of carrier oil
1 drop of peppermint ⎭

Tennis elbow

This condition, also known as lateral epicondylitis, is the most common problem affecting the forearm. The pain can be excruciating and may radiate up into the shoulder and down the whole arm and hand. Even attempting a small task such as picking up a cup or plate, opening a car door or shaking hands can induce intense pain.

'Tennis elbow' is not found only in those playing tennis, squash and other racket sports that involve repetitive arm movements, although studies reveal that 25 per cent of athletes who play once a week have suffered from it. Occupations such as typing, plastering and carpentry and leisure pursuits such as gardening, needlework and knitting can also result in this debilitating condition.

If you do play a racket sport, ensure that your racket is the right weight and size. Try to warm up and stretch your arm muscles before a game. Massage your own arms before and after playing to prevent tension from building up in the forearm. Hold your racket in your non-playing hand whenever possible.

Treatment

Tennis elbow requires rest but responds well to massage, particularly if treatment is started before the condition has become chronic. Hot and cold therapy is also effective. Elevation and compression bandaging are not required as swelling is not a problem.

Effleurage the whole arm paying particular attention to the muscles of the forearm. The primary aim of the treatment is to improve the circulation and to release adhesions and tension in the extensor muscles. Perform deep longitudinal effleurage and friction movements from the wrist to the elbow along the extensor muscles of the forearm.

It is imperative to begin treatment at the first sign of stiffness. Tennis elbow has a tendency to develop into a chronic problem, which will require anti-inflammatory medication and local steroid injections. It can even result in surgery if calcification has occurred.

Tennis elbow essential oils

1 drop of eucalyptus ⎫
1 drop of lavender   ⎬ diluted in 10 ml
1 drop of peppermint ⎭ of carrier oil

Verrucae (plantar warts)

Verrucae, or ingrowing warts, are a common problem and a nuisance for sports people. They are most often located on the sole of the foot, are highly contagious and are spread via the floors of showers, changing rooms and swimming pools where people walk barefoot. Verrucae can be extremely painful.

Treatment

Orthodox medical treatment is to cut or burn away verrucae or remove them with liquid nitrogen if they do not disappear with a proprietary wart preparation or of their own accord.

Verrucae can be effectively and simply treated with pure essential oils of lemon and tea tree. Using a cotton bud, apply undiluted a drop of either lemon or tea tree to the centre of the plantar war. Cover the area with a plaster. Repeat several times a day until the verruca disappears. This could take less than a week or up to a month. If a young child is being treated, then dilute the essential oils. Dilute one drop of tea tree and one drop of lemon into ten drops of cider vinegar.

Emergency aid

Although engaging in sports activities is highly beneficial and fairly accident-free, there are occasions where emergency first aid is required. Anyone wishing to participate in sporting activities should undertake a short first aid course such as courses taught by St John Ambulance or the Red Cross. If an accident does occur, it is vital that the correct techniques are applied immediately. Emergency aid could save a life. One of your sporting colleagues or friends could die if the appropriate action is not taken.

10

massage in the workplace

In this chapter you will learn:
- the benefits of massage at work
- how to perform a short, simple seated massage sequence in the workplace.

A rapidly increasing number of companies all over the world are realizing the benefits of massage and are heeding the call to provide massage therapy on site. Stress costs employers enormous amounts of money every year. Millions of workers are absent every workday due to stress related complaints. Numerous surveys confirm that workers perceive that they are under much more stress than ever before. Firms are curbing employee stress and absenteeism by offering heavily subsidized or even free massage treatment actually in the workplace. Increasing levels of competition and the pressure to succeed contribute to the stress in the workplace, which can have disastrous effects on our health. It is most unfortunate that so many individuals are dissatisfied with their jobs. This is hardly surprising in cases where the work environment is artificially lit, poorly ventilated, noisy and cramped. If the work is repetitive and boring and requires no skill this will also create a poor image of work. Since a major part of our life centres around our work we need to find a balance, combat our stress and enjoy our work.

Many studies have shown that a simple 10–15 minute seated massage enhances one's overall health and well-being.

Massage in the workplace:

- lowers physical stress and tension, which can lead to problems such as headaches, backache, neck and shoulder discomfort and eyestrain
- decreases blood pressure
- balances mental and emotional strain
- reduces insomnia and improves the quality of sleep
- relieves muscular and joint problems acquired during sustained or repetitive activities
- reduces tiredness and improves vitality
- stimulates the mind, increasing alertness and powers of concentration
- improves work performance
- raises staff moral and attitude so that job satisfaction is heightened and staff are positive and motivated.

An excellent, highly effective way to reduce your workplace tension is to employ the self-massage techniques described in Chapter 05. You should also follow the simple exercises outlined in Chapter 11. Try to swap an on-site chair massage regularly with your work colleagues. Some of the reasons you should consider a chair massage are:

- it's very convenient as there is no need to change clothes or shower
- it only takes 10–15 minutes – a massage can be enjoyed during the lunch or tea break
- it costs nothing
- the results are noticeable immediately
- it's easy
- it's safe
- it's both enjoyable to give as well as to receive massage.

This simple massage sequence only takes about 10 minutes and will produce excellent results.

Position for massage

Ask your partner to sit comfortably on a stool or a chair, ideally with a reasonably low back. The receiver should take off their shoes, loosen any tight clothing, uncross their legs and relax. If a cushion is available place it on the receiver's lap so that he/she can place their hands lightly on it.

You stand behind the receiver. Try to keep your back straight and distribute your weight evenly between your feet. Make sure that your neck and shoulders are relaxed and bend your knees slightly.

1 *Making contact*

To establish a connection between you and the receiver place your hands lightly onto the shoulders. Ask him/her to take a few deep breaths, allowing all the stress and tension to dissolve.

2 *Upper back – effleurage*

Place both hands, one either side of the spine, on the upper back at the level of the bottom of the shoulder blades. Gently at first and then more firmly stroke up the back around the shoulder blades and back down again. Repeat until you feel the area starting to warm up.

3 *Back – friction*

Place the balls of your thumbs level at the bottom of the shoulder blades a few centimetres away from the spine. Perform small, slow deep circular friction movements working towards the neck area. Do NOT press directly onto the spine itself.

If you find any 'knotty' areas friction over these nodules until you feel them breaking down or the discomfort subsides.

4 Shoulder blades – *effleurage*

Stand to the side of the receiver. If you are treating the right scapula you should position yourself on the left hand side, place your left arm over the front of the shoulders and your right hand, palm down on the right scapula. Circle around the shoulder blade until you feel the area warm and soften. Repeat on the other side.

5 Shoulder blade – *rubbing*

In the same position as step 4, use the whole of your hand to rub across the scapula. Repeat on the other side.

6 Shoulder blade – *friction*

Still in the same position place your thumb at the bottom of the scapula and apply deep circular movements all around the shoulder blade.

7 Shoulders – *squeezing*

Stand behind the receiver and place the palms of both hands, one on top of each shoulder with your thumbs at the back and fingers at the front. Squeeze and release the shoulder muscles until they feel warm.

8 Shoulders – *wringing*

Standing behind your partner place the palms of both hands on top of one of the shoulders. Pick up and squeeze the muscle with one hand and pull it towards you and then repeat with the other hand. Repeat the wringing on both shoulders until they feel soft and supple.

9 Arms – *squeezing*

Still standing behind the receiver place the hands one on each upper arm. Gently squeeze and release the muscles, working down the upper arms towards the elbow and glide gently back again. Repeat several times.

10 Neck – *squeezing*

Stand to the side of your partner. Let their forehead drop slightly forwards into one hand and place your other hand flat on the back of the neck. Squeeze the neck muscles slowly and gently between your thumb and fingers.

11 Head – *making contact*

Standing behind the receiver place your hands softly on top of the receiver's head to establish a connection.

12 Scalp – friction
Place your hands either side of the head, with the fingers well spread out in a claw shape. Use the pads of your fingers to make small circular friction movements over the whole of the scalp. As the tension releases you will feel the scalp starting to move.

13 Face – effleurage
Standing behind the receiver place the palms of your hands gently on the forehead. Stroke gently out across the forehead towards the temples. Then place your hands on the cheeks and stroke outwards and finally stroke outwards across the chin.

Repeat these wonderfully soothing movements several times.

14 The wake up!
Positioned behind the receiver use your fingertips to gently drum/tap all over the head. Try experimenting with different rhythms. You may also lightly tap all over the face too. This gentle tapping helps to stimulate and energize the mind ready for the rest of the working day!

If you are interested in learning more movements for the shoulders, neck and head refer to *Teach Yourself Indian Head Massage* by the same author.

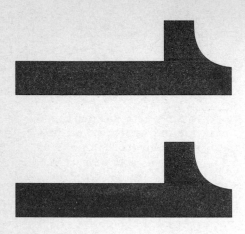

a healthy lifestyle

In this chapter you will learn:
- the importance of massage througout every stage of life
- recommendations for a healthy diet
- exercises to keep your body strong, supple and fit.

A healthy body requires regular massage, a healthy diet and daily exercise. This chapter tells you how to achieve optimum health and fitness.

Massage

Massage is vital for our physical, emotional and spiritual well-being. It is beneficial for all of us throughout the various stages of life.

Massage of the newborn helps the child's physiological and emotional development. Babies and children of all ages who receive regular massage therapy will not only feed and sleep much better, but are also far less prone to health problems. They also derive a great deal of pleasure from being massaged.

During the traumatic period of adolescence, massage can bridge the 'generation gap' between teenagers and adults. Touch can help to minimize stress and tension within the family unit, helps to stabilize behavioural problems and regulates hormonal imbalances.

If massage is performed before sporting activities the likelihood of muscle strains is decreased considerably and performance, stamina and agility will be enhanced. When minor sports injuries are sustained, massage is a highly effective treatment and provides an excellent aid to recuperation.

Massage in the workplace reduces stress and tension, relieves muscular and joint problems, banishes insomnia, increases alertness and work performance and raises staff morale so that we are positive and motivated.

Massage can help a woman throughout the enormous physical and emotional changes of pregnancy and prepares her for childbirth. It provides a gentle way to relieve the minor discomforts associated with pregnancy without undesirable side effects. The mother-to-be experiences deep relaxation, an improved sleep pattern and a boost in energy levels. Back pain, mood swings, fluid retention, varicose veins, aching legs and cramps, headaches and stretch marks may all be prevented.

Massage therapy during the menopause enables a woman to adapt physically and emotionally to this enormous 'change' in life. On an emotional level it helps to lift depression, balances mood swings and dispels irrational thoughts and feelings of insecurity and low self-esteem. On a physical level hot flushes, headaches, fluctuations in energy, fluid retention and weight gain can all be treated naturally with massage, essential oils, diet and exercise.

In later life massage is a wonderful way of enhancing the quality of life. The pain, stiffness and lack of mobility that accompanies arthritis and rheumatism can be considerably reduced. The flexibility of muscles and joints improves. Circulation is stimulated and toxins are cleansed from the system far more efficiently. The texture and tone of the skin improves, digestion and elimination are more effective, and depression and anxiety are much less prevalent.

Thus, throughout all the stages of life massage has a vital role to play and has something to offer everyone. When combined with a healthy diet and regular exercise it promotes increased energy and vitality, suppleness, relaxation, peace of mind and happiness.

Healthy diet

Let food be your medicine, and let medicine be your food.
Hippocrates

A good diet is essential for our health and well-being. Poor nutrition combined with excessive stress, drugs, pollution and a lack of exercise will inevitably lead to a compromised level of health and ultimately to serious disease.

Often individuals are completely unaware that they are operating below par because they have never experienced what it is like to feel healthy. They are accustomed to accepting their three colds every year, mysterious 'viruses', monthly, weekly or even daily headaches, irregular bowel movements, aching muscles and stiff, painful creaking joints. They expect to get extreme fatigue as a result of coping with the stresses and strains of modern life. Such individuals are opening up their bodies to the likelihood of more serious illnesses. Often it is only after the appearance of serious disease that an individual can be persuaded to change his or her diet. Eating habits are formed early in life and it is always so much easier to continue with old patterns of nutrition than it is to change. However, once a person has made the initial effort the benefits of the new nutritional régime rapidly become apparent.

A healthy balanced diet helps you to repair the damage to your body which may be the result of years of abuse. Regard it as an 'insurance policy' to promote good health. Prevention is always preferable to cure.

Guidelines for a healthy diet

For most people the ideal diet should consist of 70–80 per cent alkaline forming foods and only 20–30 per cent acid forming foods. The principal alkaline forming foods are fresh fruits and vegetables. Acid forming foods include all meat, grains, cheese, eggs, fish, coffee and tea.

Too much acid causes disease – the overproduction of mucus, tension in the nervous system, arthritis, rheumatism, respiratory problems, digestive disorders and so on. A high intake of alkaline forming foods can improve your health enormously.

If you do decide to change your diet, don't try to do it all at once. Change **slowly**. Dietary changes should never be drastic, otherwise too many toxins are released into the bloodstream making you feel uncomfortable and ill. Tackle one problem at a time – take one item, such as sugar, and eliminate it. Do not become too fanatical about what you eat. Try to follow these recommendations:

- Increase your intake of fresh fruit. Fruit is a major source of vitamin C and contains many other vitamins, minerals and fibre. It is also low in fat and low in calories. Fruits are alkaline and excellent cleansers, especially apples, pears and grapes.
- Increase your daily intake of fresh vegetables especially green leafy vegetables. Vegetables are low in fat and calories, provide us with fibre and are rich in vitamins and minerals. Raw or lightly cooked green vegetables or salads are particularly nutritious. Cooking destroys some of the nutrients, especially vitamin C. You should aim to have **at least** five portions of fruit and/or vegetables daily.
- Eat more fibre – beans, pulses, cereals, such as wheat, oats, barley, corn, rice and rye (especially wholegrain) and fruits and vegetables. A diet high in fibre reduces constipation and other bowel problems and certain forms of cancer.
- Reduce your intake of refined carbohydrates and sugar. These are 'empty calories' containing little or no nutrition. Avoid sweets, cakes, biscuits, jams, marmalades, chocolates and fizzy drinks or squashes. Always check the label ingredients for sugar content.
- Moderate your fat intake, especially **saturated** fat, which is associated with heart disease. If you eat meat buy only lean meat, and try to eat more fish. Cut down on high fat foods such as pastries, pies, sausages, preserved and tinned meats.

Take dairy foods sparingly. Grill foods rather than frying them. When cooking choose an oil high in unsaturates such as vegetable and seed oils.

- Reduce your salt intake in cooking and in foods. High intakes are associated with high blood pressure.
- Moderate your alcohol consumption.
- Avoid chemical additives, such as preservatives and colouring. Eat fresh foods whenever possible.
- Reduce your caffeine intake in coffee, tea and cola.
- Take care with food combinations – try not to have protein and starch together at the same meal. Starch requires alkaline conditions for digestion whereas protein requires acid conditions. Both cannot be produced at the same time. Acid and alkaline neutralize each other, so if you eat both protein and starch together neither will be properly digested. This system of eating is known as 'food combining' or the 'Hay Diet'.
- When cooking use only pottery, stainless steel, iron or glass. Never use bare aluminium, which is toxic to the nervous system. One pre-senile dementia (Alzheimer's disease) has been linked with a high level of aluminium in the brain. Aluminium can also accumulate in the liver and affect the kidneys.
- Avoid smoking, which has many harmful effects.
- Take medical drugs only if essential.
- Take regular physical exercise which is vital to good health. Try to have a brisk walk daily.
- Think positively! Positive emotions such as love, hope and laughter can block out the negative emotions such as fear and panic. Emotional nutrients such as love are vital for optimum health.

Exercise

Eating properly will not by itself keep well a person who does not exercise, for food and exercise, being opposite in effect, work together to produce health.

Hippocrates

Exercise is vital to good health and will enable you to keep your body strong, supple and fit. The exercises described below are simple and will help to prevent muscular and joint problems from occurring. If you find it diffcult to exercise at home I strongly recommend you join a Yoga class (see 'Useful addresses', p.188).

Exercises for the back

The majority of the population will suffer from back pain of some description at some time in their lives. In fact, over 30 million working days are lost each year as a result of bad backs. However, if we keep our backs healthy with regular exercise and massage and we improve our posture to minimize the strain on the joints and soft tissues, many back problems will be avoided. The following remedial exercises are designed to help your spine to regain strength and flexibility. Try to make this exercise programme part of your daily routine. Always perform the exercises **slowly** avoiding any quick, jerky movements and never overstretch and overstrain. If you experience sharp pains while doing these exercises, stop at once and consult your doctor or osteopath.

Find a comfortable place to exercise and place a blanket, mat or thick towel on the floor. While exercising it is important to breathe deeply – never hold your breath. Take a few deep breaths before you begin. Place both hands on your abdomen just below your naval and breathe in. As you inhale, your abdomen should rise as it fills with air. As you exhale your abdomen should fall.

Exercise 1 – The pelvic tilt

Lie on your back with your knees bent up, and your feet apart and flat on the floor. Place your hands down on the small of your back and feel the arch in your lower back. In this exercise you will try to press this arch down to meet the floor. Squeeze your buttocks together, tighten the muscles of your abdomen and then raise your buttocks slightly off the floor (see Figure 11.1). Hold this position for a count of ten. Relax. Repeat three times.

Benefits
The pelvic tilt will reduce the stress on your lower back and tighten your abdominals and buttocks.

Exercise 2 – Knees to the chest

One knee
Lying on the floor as in Exercise 1, clasp both hands around your right knee and slowly bring it towards your chest (see Figure 11.2). Hold this position for ten seconds. Gently allow your leg to return to the original position. Repeat this exercise with the left knee. Repeat three times in total.

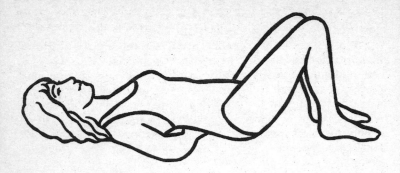

figure 11.1   the pelvic tilt

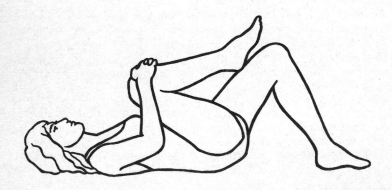

figure 11.2   knees to the chest

Both knees

Bring your right knee and then your left towards your chest. Clasp both hands around your knees and pull your knees down towards your chest, as close as you can. Hold this position for a count of ten. Return to the starting position and repeat three times.

Benefits

The muscles in both your hips and buttocks are given a good stretch.

Exercise 3 – The gentle trunk twister

Place the hands clasped underneath your head with the elbows outstretched at right angles. Bring the knees up and slowly cross your right leg over the left thigh. Allow the weight of your right leg to slowly push the left knee towards the floor. As you do so slowly turn the head towards the right shoulder. Hold this position for ten seconds. Ensure that your shoulders remain flat on the floor throughout the exercise. Only stretch as far as it is comfortable. Gently return to the starting position. Repeat on the opposite side, crossing the left knee over the right thigh and turning the head towards the left shoulder.

Benefits

The lower back and abdominal muscles are stretched and strengthened. Flexibility of the spine is encouraged.

Exercise 4 – The cobra

This is an exercise based on yoga with wonderful therapeutic effects. Lie face down. Place both hands in front of you palms downwards just below the shoulders. Breathe in deeply slowly raising your head back as far as you can and using your arms push the chest slowly away from the floor so that the whole spine curves back. Hold this position for seven seconds ensuring that the stomach is pressed firmly against the floor. Slowly return to the starting position.

Benefits

The lower back is strengthened and posture is improved.

Exercise 5 – The cat

This is another yoga exercise. Kneel down on your hands and knees in a crawling position with the hands shoulder width apart and the knees approximately eight inches apart. Keeping your arms and legs still slowly arch your back to hump it upwards lowering your head and tucking the chin into the chest. Hold this position for seven seconds.

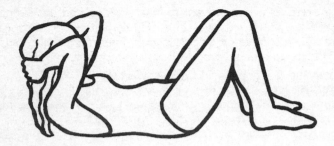

figure 11.3   partial sit-ups

Exercise for the abdomen

It is important to strengthen the abdominal muscles. Weak abdominal muscles will cause back pain disturbing the balance between the erector spinae muscle group and the abdominals. Weak abdominal muscles create bad posture – the abdomen protrudes and the lumbar spine curves too far inwards. The abdominal muscles are also essential for supporting the internal organs. Weakness can lead to problems with the bowels and the reproductive organs.

Partial sit-ups

Lie on your back with your knees bent up and your feet apart and flat on the floor. You can either place your arms at your sides or clasp your hands underneath your head.

Tuck your chin on to your chest and slowly raise both your head and shoulders off the floor. Hold this position for seven seconds. Lower yourself back to the floor. Repeat three times.

Benefits
Your abdominal muscles will be strengthened and toned. Your internal organs will be supported and massaged.

Exercises for the legs

Leg exercises are important for maintaining and increasing the flexibility of the legs and hips. The legs must be warmed up before any sporting activity to avoid injury. Exercising the legs also helps to reduce fatty deposits around the hips and thighs.

Exercise 1 – The hurdler's stretch
Sit on the floor. Stretch your right leg straight out in front of you with your knee pressed firmly into the ground and your foot dorsiflexed (pulled upwards). Bend your left knee up and tuck it sideways out of the way. Slowly and carefully bend forwards as far as you can without causing any pain (see Figure 11.4). Hold this position for ten seconds.

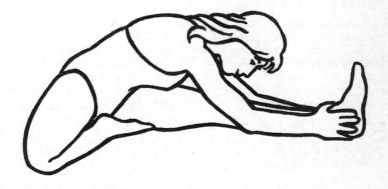

figure 11.4 the hurdler's stretch

Repeat this stretching movement on the other side. Repeat three times.

Benefits

This exercise stretches your hamstring muscles in the back of your thigh. It also increases flexibility of your knees. The hamstrings are particularly under stress when sprinting, playing football and karate kicking. If your hamstrings are taut then you will have difficulty touching your toes.

Exercise 2 – The half lunge

Stand up facing a wall. Place the palms of your hands shoulder width apart against the wall.

Place the right leg straight behind you in a lunge position. The left leg remains forward and is flexed. Push gently against the feet feeling the stretch in the legs. Hold this position for ten seconds.

Come back slowly to the starting position and repeat the exercise on the other leg.

Benefits

Increases flexibility of the legs, hamstrings and hips. Aids the reduction of fatty deposits around the hips and thighs. An excellent warm up exercise prior to sporting activities.

Exercise 3 – The sitting stretch

Sit on the floor with the legs straight out in front of you. Keeping your back as straight as possible reach forward slowly aiming to try to reach your ankles or feet with your hands. Hold this position for ten seconds.

Benefits

This exercise also stretches and increases flexibility

Exercise 4 – The squat

Standing up place the feet shoulder width apart. Tighten up both the abdominal and the buttock muscles. With the back straight and the arms stretched out in front of you slowly lower yourself as far as possible into the squatting position (if you find it difficult to balance then hold on to a chair). Hold this position for seven seconds and then gradually return to your original position.

Repeat this exercise three times.

Benefits

The squatting exercise is particularly good for strengthening the thighs and buttocks. It also improves balance and posture.

Exercises for the feet

Foot exercises will keep the feet healthy, supple and flexible. They also alleviate and disperse any fluid that may have collected around the ankles, and improve the circulation.

Foot mobility

1 Pick up a pencil with your toes. Hold it for a count of five and then put it down again. Repeat ten times.
2 Sitting down dorsiflex your foot and plantar flex your foot ten times.
3 With your foot relaxed turn your ankle round ten times in circles clockwise and anticlockwise.

Exercises for the neck

Your neck should be able to move freely forwards, backwards and sideways. Most people, however, find that movement is limited in at least one direction and all of us will suffer at least once in our lives from a stiff neck.

When performing neck exercises always stop immediately if symptoms such as dizziness occur. Never force movements and always perform them slowly and carefully.

Neck mobilization

1 Sitting or standing, slowly and gently bend your head forwards so that your chin ideally touches your sternum (breastbone). Then lift your chin up until the back of your head touches your neck. Repeat about five times.
2 Turn your head gently and slowly from side to side. Repeat about five times.
3 Incline your head to one side attempting to touch your ear to your shoulder and then incline your head to the other side. Repeat approximately five times.

Exercises for the shoulders

The shoulder joint is the most mobile joint in the body. A whole host of movements is possible – flexion, extension, abduction, adduction, rotation and circumduction.

Always be wary of pains without a recognizable cause in the left shoulder radiating down the left arm which appear on exertion. These should be checked out by a medical practitioner in case they suggest a heart condition.

The majority of us have an enormous number of knots and nodules in our shoulders. It is a major area for the accumulation of stress and tension – hence the expression 'carrying the weight of the world upon the shoulders'. Most occupations also put a great deal of strain on the shoulders – leaning forwards over a desk, computer or typewriter, performing repetitive, awkward, often one-sided movements and so forth. You should keep to a daily routine of shoulder exercises.

Shoulder mobilization
1 *Towel stretch*
Standing with your legs apart, with your elbows straight, hold a towel in both hands in front of you. Slowly swing your arms back over your head, keeping the towel taut and then swing back to your original position. Repeat ten times.

2 *Clapping*
Standing with your legs apart, keeping your elbows straight, swing your arms forwards and backwards clapping your hands both in front of your chest and behind your back. Repeat 20 times.

3 *Circumduction*
Standing with your arms in a relaxed position hanging at your sides, circle your right arm slowly ten times in both directions. Repeat with the left arm.

Exercises for the wrists and hands
Our hands are used constantly and repetitively in our daily activities. Exercise can promote strength and mobility.

Exercise 1 – Strengthening
Squeeze a squash ball for a count of five, as hard as you can, then stretch out your fingers. Repeat ten times with each hand.

Exercise 2 – Strengthening
Place your hands flat on a table with your palms down. Spread your fingers out sideways as far as possible, and then bring them together again, keeping your fingers in close contact with the table.

Exercise 3 – Mobilizing the fingers
With your hands flat on a table, palms down and your fingers slightly spread, lift each finger in turn, take it to each side and lower. The other fingers should remain as still as possible. Repeat ten times.

Basic anatomy

I will try to keep the bones and muscles of the body as easy to understand as possible. Muscles appear very complex at first but, in fact, are simple and logical to learn. As we will be massaging the muscles it is advisable to know what the muscles are called and what they actually do. Below is useful terminology for describing the action of muscles:

flexion where a forward or anterior movement of the limb or trunk occurs

extension where a backward or posterior movement of the limb occurs

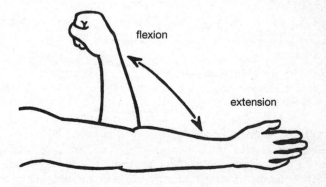

abduction where a limb moves away from the middle of the body
adduction where a limb moves towards the middle of the body or returns to its original position

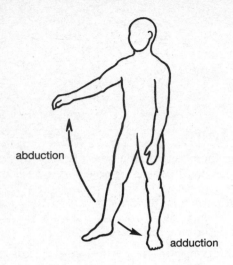

abduction

adduction

pronation where the palm is turned downwards
supination where the palm is turned upwards

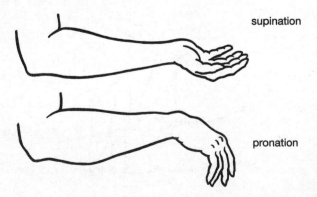

supination

pronation

medial rotation where a limb is rotated towards the midline of the body
lateral rotation where a limb is rotated away from the midline of the body

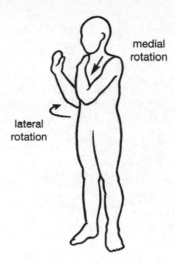

medial
rotation

lateral
rotation

circumduction drawing a circle in space

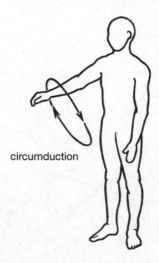

circumduction

inversion where the sole of the foot is turned inwards
eversion where the sole of the foot is turned outwards

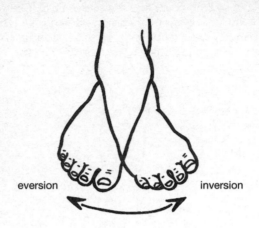

eversion   inversion

dorsiflexion where the foot is pulled back
plantar flexion where the foot is pointed

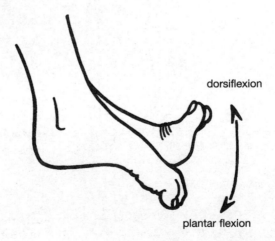

dorsiflexion

plantar flexion

The leg

The main bones of the leg are:

Below the knee

1 The **tibia** in the lower leg known as the 'shin' bone, the larger bone of the lower leg, is situated medially and is involved with the knee joint at the top and with the ankle joint at the bottom. It articulates with the **femur** and the **fibula**. The medial (inside) surface of the lower end of the tibia forms the medial malleolus.

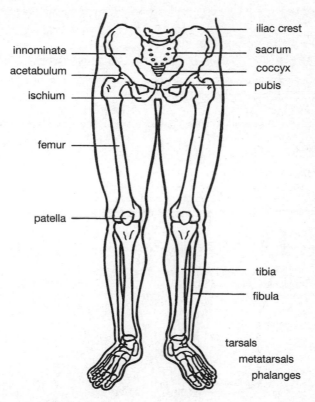

bones of the leg and pelvis

2 The **fibula,** also in the lower leg, is a much thinner bone situated laterally. It articulates with the tibia and forms part of the ankle joint. The lower end of the fibula forms the lateral malleolus.

Above the knee

3 The **femur** (thighbone) is the largest bone of the lower limb. It forms the thigh and is the longest and heaviest bone of the body. It has a rounded upper end called the head, which fits into a deep cup-shaped socket known as the acetabulum and forms the hip joint.

The lower end of the femur has two condyles (rounded ends) called the medial condyle and the lateral condyle for articulation with the tibia.

The knee cap is a small triangular bone known as the **patella**.

Muscles of the lower leg

The **posterior** muscles of the lower leg (calf muscles) include:

1 The **gastrocnemius** (gaster=belly kneme=leg) is the most superficial muscle of the calf and has two heads.

    Origin – back of the leg, just above the knee

    Insertion – via the Achilles tendon into the calcaneus (heel bone)

    Function – the action of the gastrocnemius is to plantar flex the foot

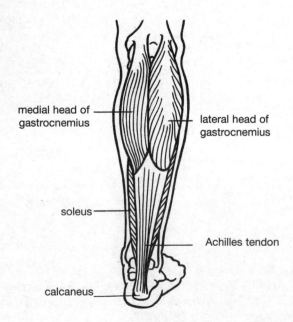

muscles of the back of the lower leg

2 The **soleus** (soleus=sole of the foot) lies deep to the gastrocnemius.
Origin – tibia and fibula
Insertion – via the Achilles tendon into the calcaneus
Function – the soleus also plantar flexes the foot

3 The **tibialis posterior** (posterior=back, tibialis=tibia)
Origin – back of the tibia and fibula
Insertion – medial tarsal and metatarsal bones
Function – plantar flexes and inverts the foot

The tibialis posterior is also very important for supporting the medial longitudinal arch of the foot and weakness will cause 'rolling' of the feet inwards.

N.B: The posterior calf muscles of the leg are **all** involved in **plantar flexion** of the ankle. Other flexor muscles include the **flexor digitorum longus** (long flexor muscle of the toes), which flexes the toes, and plantar flexes the foot and the **flexor hallucis longus** (long flexor muscle of the big toe), which flexes the big toe and assists plantar flexion of the foot.

The **anterior** muscles of the lower leg includes the **tibialis anterior** (anterior=front, tibialis=tibia) which is the largest muscle on the front of the leg and can easily be palpated.
Origin – outer side of the tibia just below the knee
Insertion – inner edge of the foot, towards the big toe (medial cuneiform and first metatarsal).

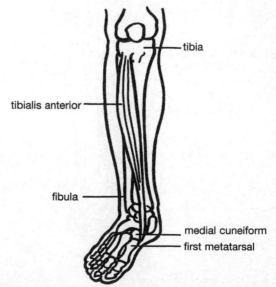

tibialis anterior

Function – dorsiflexes the foot and inverts the foot. The tibialis anterior (like the tibialis posterior) is also important for maintaining the medial longitudinal arch of the foot and prevents the foot from 'rolling' inwards.

Other muscles include the **extensor digitorum longus** (long extensor muscle of the toes), which extends from the upper two-thirds of the anterior surface of the fibula to the four toes. This muscle dorsiflexes the foot and extends the toes. The **extensor hallucis longus** (long extensor muscle of the big toe) arises from the middle half of the anterior surface of the fibula inserting into the big toe. It extends the great toe and assists with dorsiflexion of the foot.

The **lateral** (outside) muscles of the lower leg include: the **peroneus longus** and **peroneus brevis** (perone=fibula, longus=long, brevis=short).

Origin – outer side of the leg attached to the fibula
Insertion – the peroneus longus is attached to the first metatarsal, the peroneus brevis is attached to the fifth metatarsal
Function – plantar flexes and everts the foot

The **peroneal** muscles are also important for giving lateral sideways stability for the ankle and will prevent the feet from 'rolling' outwards.

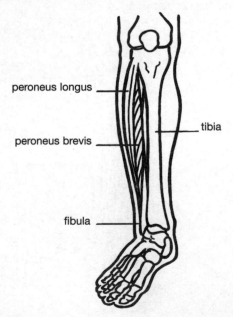

peroneus longus

tibia

peroneus brevis

fibula

peroneal muscles

Muscles of the upper leg

The **posterior** muscles of the upper leg (back of the thigh) include:

The **hamstrings** (hamme=back of the leg, stringere=to draw together) are composed of three muscles, namely:

1 **biceps** (two heads) **femoris** is located towards the lateral aspect (outside) of the thigh
2 **semitendinosus** (semi=half, tendo=tendon) ⎤ located towards
3 **semimembranosus** (semi=half, ⎬ the medial aspect
   membran=membrane) ⎦ (inside) of the thigh

Origin – ischial tuberosity (bottom of the pelvis). The short head of the biceps femoris arises from the lower back part of the femur
Insertion – either side of the tibia
Function – the hamstrings flex the knee and extend the thigh

If there are problems with the hamstrings then there may be a problem with the pelvis that requires manipulation by a qualified osteopath.

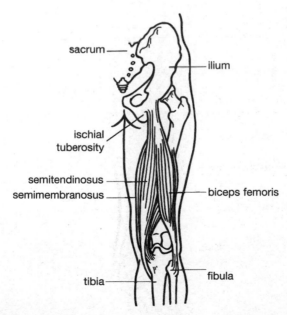

hamstrings

The **anterior** muscles of the upper leg (front of the thigh) include:

1 The **quadriceps femoris** (quad=four, caput=head, femoris=femur) are composed of four muscles, namely:

i) **rectus femoris** (rectus=fibres parallel to the midline)
ii) **vastus lateralis** (vastus=large)
iii) **vastus intermedius**
iv) **vastus medialis**

> Origin – all the vastus muscles originate from the upper part of the femur. The rectus femoris originates from the front part of the **ilium**
> Insertion – through the patella and on to the tibia
> Function – all four quadriceps extend the knee and the rectus femoris flexes the thigh

If there are problems with the quadriceps then there will be great difficulty trying to straighten the knee.

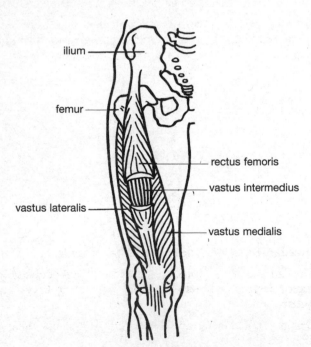

quadriceps

2 The **sartorius** (sartor=tailor) is often referred to as the 'tailor's muscle' since it is used when you sit cross-legged as tailors used to.

Origin – ilium
Insertion – medial aspect (inside) of the tibia
Function – flexes the knee and the hip and abducts the thigh and rotates the thigh laterally

If the sartorius muscle is weak then knee problems will result, particularly on the inside of the knee, possibly causing knock knees.

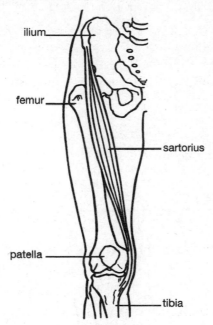

ilium

femur

sartorius

patella

tibia

sartorius

The **medial** (inner) muscles of the thigh include:

1 The **adductors** (ad=to, ducere=to bring) consist of the **adductor longus, adductor magnus, adductor brevis** and the **pectineus**.

Origin – pubic bone and lower half of the hip bone (ischial tuberosity)
Insertion – inside of the femur
Function – adduction of the thigh and lateral rotation of the thigh

If the adductors are weak there will be difficulty in locking the knees. Groin strains in these muscles are common.

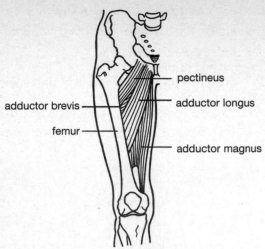

adductors

2 The **gracilis** (gracilis=slender)

Origin – pubic bone
Insertion – inside of the tibia (upper part)
Function – adduction of the thigh. Medial rotation of the thigh. Flexes the leg.

If the gracilis is weak this can lead to 'knock knee' problems.

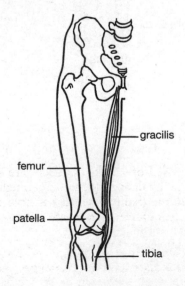

gracilis

The **lateral** (outer) muscles of the thigh include:

The **tensor fasciae latae** (tensor = makes tense, latus = wide)

Origin – outer edge of the iliac crest
Insertion – outside of the tibia
Function – abduction and medial rotation of the thigh. Flexes the thigh

The tensor fasciae latae is an enormous muscle, which often becomes very tense (hypertonic) resulting in pelvic problems and also knee pain.

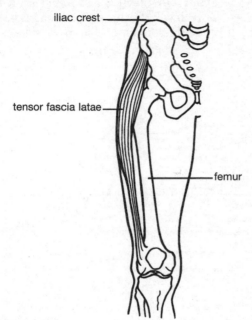

tensor fasciae latae

The foot

Each foot is composed of 26 bones. There are 14 **phalanges** – each toe has three phalanges (distal, intermediate, proximal) apart from the big toe (hallux) which has only two phalanges. The phalanges articulate with each other and with the **metatarsals**.

There are five metatarsals – one metatarsal bone for each toe. The metatarsals articulate with the phalanges and the **tarsals**.

There are seven **tarsal** bones, namely:
    calcaneus
    talus
    cuboid
    navicular
    First **cuneiform** (medial)
    Second **cuneiform** (intermediate)
    Third **cuneiform** (lateral)

The **calcaneus** and **talus** are located on the posterior part of the foot. The calcaneus is the largest and strongest of the tarsal bones. The talus articulates with the tibia and fibula at the ankle joint. The talus has the medial malleolus of the tibia on one side and the lateral malleolus of the fibula on the other side.

The **cuboid**, **navicular** and the three **cuneiform** bones are located on the anterior part of the foot.

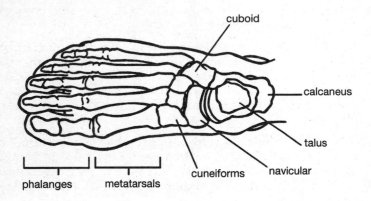

The bones of the foot are arranged to produce distinct arches, which allow the foot to support the weight of the body. These arches are springy, yielding as the weight of the body is applied to the ground and springing back as weight is lifted.

1 Medial (inner) longitudinal arch – formed by the calcaneus, navicular, three cuneiform and the medial three metarsal bones. This is the highest of the arches and only the calcaneus and the distal end of the metatarsals should touch the ground.
2 Lateral (outer) longitudinal arch – formed by the calcaneus, cuboid and the two lateral metatarsal bones. This arch is lower and less mobile than the medial longitudinal arch.

3 Transverse arches (running across the foot) – formed by the metatarsals, the three cuneiforms, cuboid and navicular. The bones of the foot are held in position by strong ligaments and leg muscle tendons. If these are weakened then the arches will flatten, resulting in a condition called 'fallen arches' or 'flat foot'.

The back

The spine, or vertebral column, is composed of 26 **vertebrae**, which are distributed as follows:

seven **cervical vertebrae** (cervix=neck)
twelve **thoracic/dorsal vertebrae**
five **lumbar vertebrae** (lumbus=loin)
one **sacrum** (five sacral vertebrae fused together)
one **coccyx** (four vetebrae fused together)

Therefore, before the fusion of the sacral and coccygeal vertebrae the total number of vertebrae is 33.

Between adjacent vertebrae are the **intervertebral discs**. These discs have a shock-absorbing function, and the joints that they form allow movements of the vertebral column. They consist of an outer rim of fibrocartilage called the **annulus fibrosis** and an inner soft, pulpy, gelatinous material called the **nucleus pulposus**.

When viewed from the side the vertebral column presents four curves. These curves are important as they increase the strength of the vertebral column, make balance possible in the upright position, protect the column from fracture and absorb any jars when walking.

Muscles of the back and shoulders

1 The **erector spinae** (*sacrospinalis*)

The erector muscles of the spine consists of three groupings:

iliocostalis (laterally placed)
longissimus (intermediately placed)
spinalis (medially placed)

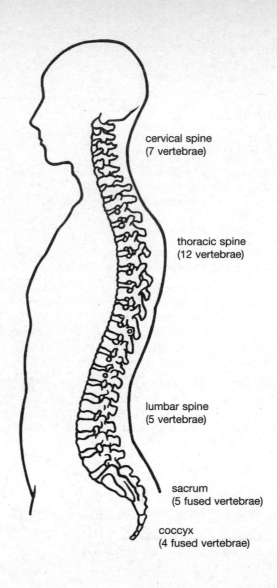

cervical spine
(7 vertebrae)

thoracic spine
(12 vertebrae)

lumbar spine
(5 vertebrae)

sacrum
(5 fused vertebrae)

coccyx
(4 fused vertebrae)

vertebral column

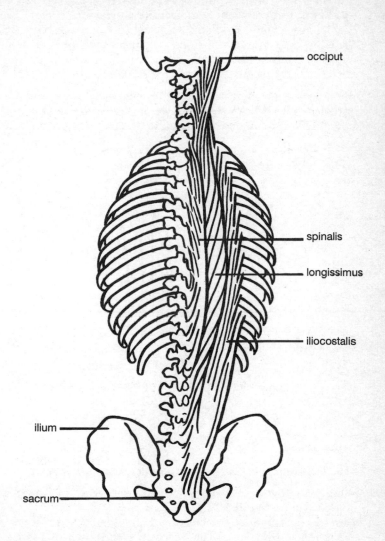

occiput

spinalis

longissimus

iliocostalis

ilium

sacrum

erector spinae (sacrospinalis)

These groups consist of a series of overlapping muscle. It runs along each side of the vertebral column.

Origin – crest of the ilium, sacrum, vertebrae and ribs
Insertion – ribs, vertebrae, occiput (base of skull)
Function – extension of the spine when both sides contract (backbending); lateral flexion (sidebending) of the spine when one side contracts; maintenance of the erect posture of the trunk: acting singly the erector spinae rotates the trunk

If one side is in spasm it will often protrude like a rope down the contracted side. If both sides are weak then the individual will slouch and will be unable to maintain an erect posture.

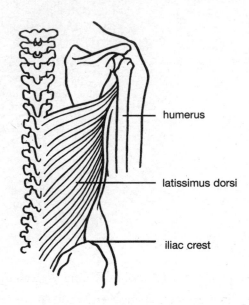

latissimus dorsi

2 The **latissimus dorsi** (latissimus=widest, dorsum=back)

Origin – lower six thoracic vertebrae, the five lumbar vertebrae and the iliac crest
Insertion – humerus just below the shoulder
Function – draws the arm backwards and inwards towards the body

3 The **serratus anterior** (serra=saw, anterior=front)

Origin – upper eight or nine ribs
Insertion – scapula (medial border nearest the spine)
Function – draws the scapula forwards and rotates it

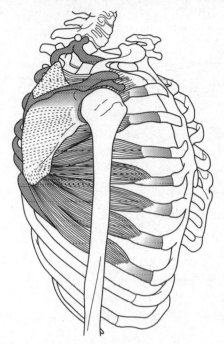

serratus anterior

4 The **trapezius** (trapezoides=trapezoid shape)

Origin – occiput, cervical and thoracic vertebrae
Insertion – clavicle (collar bone) and spine of the scapula
Function – elevates or lowers the scapula, rotates scapula,
adducts scapula, rotates and bends the head backward

The **trapezius** is the most superficial of all the muscles of the upper back and neck. Tension and stiffness of this muscle result in upper back and neck problems and pain between the shoulder blades. Headaches may also arise from tension in the trapezius muscle. Problems in this area are often related to poor posture such as slouching while relaxing in a chair.

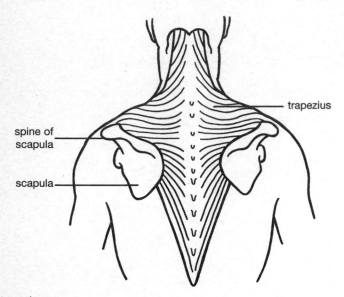

spine of scapula

scapula

trapezius

trapezius

5 The **deltoid** (delta=triangular)

Origin – clavicle and the spine of the scapula
Insertion – side of the humerus about halfway down
Function – abduction of the arm; assists in flexion and extension of the arm

6 The **supraspinatus** (supra=above, spinatus=spine of the scapula)

Origin – above the spine of the scapula
Insertion – top of the humerus
Function – abduction of the arm

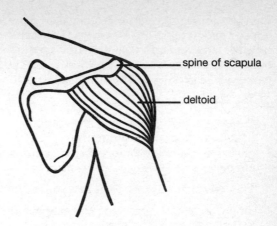

deltoid

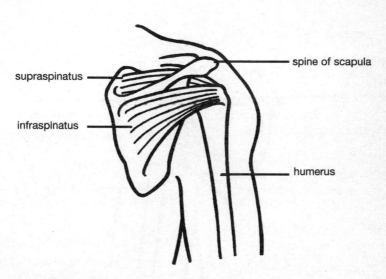

supraspinatus and infraspinatus

Damage to this muscle is a common cause of shoulder pain which may even radiate down the arm. Sports requiring repetitive movements with the arm raised above the shoulder such as racket sports and crawl and backstroke in swimming can result in problems with this muscle.

7 The **infraspinatus** (infra=below)

Origin – below the spine of the scapula
Insertion – top of the humerus
Function – lateral rotation of the arm (together with the teres minor).

8 The **teres minor** (teres=long and round, minor=small)

Origin – lateral border of the scapula (i.e. the side of the scapula closest to the arm)
Insertion – top of the humerus
Function – lateral rotation of the arm (together with the infraspinatus)

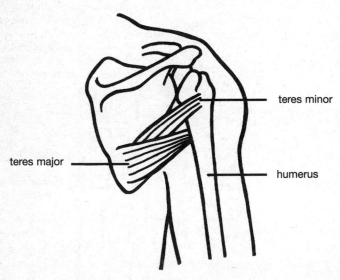

teres minor and teres major

The infraspinatus and the teres minor work closely together. Pain from these muscles makes it difficult to rotate the arm inwards and also to reach across the back to touch the other shoulder.

9 The **teres major** (teres=long and round)

Origin – bottom lateral edge of the scapula
Insertion – back of the humerus
Function – medial rotation and adduction of the arm, extension of the shoulder joint

10 The greater and lesser **rhomboids** (rhomboides=rhomboid or diamond-shaped)

Origin – seventh cervical vertebra and the first five thoracic vertebrae
Insertion – medial border of the scapula
Function – adduction of the scapula (pulling back the shoulder blades)

Pain and tension can develop in these muscles as a result of poor posture. Occupational stress such as working behind a desk all day may also cause discomfort between the shoulder blades.

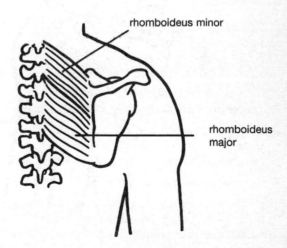

rhomboids

The levator scapulae (levator=lifter)

Origin – first four cervical vertebrae

Insertion – top of the scapula

Function – elevates (raises) the scapula. If the scapula is fixed, it side bends the neck.

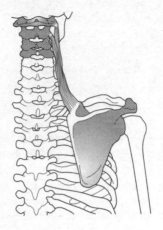

levator scapulae

Muscles of the buttocks

The **gluteals** are composed of the **gluteus maximus** (glutos=buttock, maximus=largest), the **gluteus medius** (media=middle) and the **gluteus minimus** (minimus=smallest).

1 The gluteus maximus (largest muscle of the buttocks)

Origin – back of the ilium, sacrum and coccyx

Insertion – top back of the femur

Function – lateral rotation of the thigh; extension of the hip

2 Gluteus medius/gluteus minimus

Origin – ilium

Insertion – top of the side of the femur

Function – abduction of the thigh; the gluteus minimus assists in lateral rotation of the thigh; the gluteus medius rotates the thigh medially

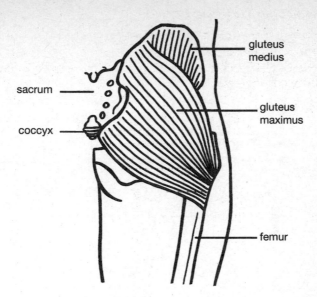

gluteals

Excessive tension in the gluteal muscles often results in low back problems.

The arm and hand

The **humerus** is the upper bone of the arm and the head articulates with the **glenoid** cavity of the scapula to form the shoulder joint. Deep muscles of the shoulder and their tendons strengthen and stabilise the shoulder joint. The distal end of the humerus articulates with the **radius** and the **ulna** (the two bones of the forearm) to form the elbow joint. The ulna is the medial bone of the forearm – in other words it is found at the little finger side. The radius is the lateral bone of the forearm – it is situated on the thumb side. The radius and ulna also articulate with the **carpal** bones or wrist bones. The carpus (wrist) consists of eight bones arranged in two rows, namely:

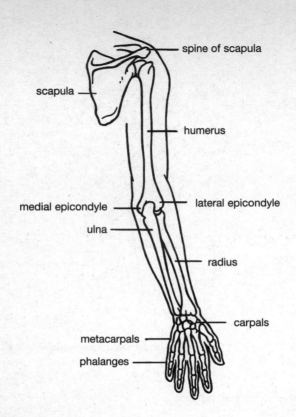

spine of scapula

scapula

humerus

medial epicondyle

lateral epicondyle

ulna

radius

carpals

metacarpals

phalanges

bones of the arm and hand

scaphoid
lunate
triquetral
pisiform
} first row

trapezium
trapezoid
capitate
hamate
} second row

There are five **metacarpals**, one for each finger, which form the framework of the palm of the hand.

There are fourteen **phalanges** or finger bones – two phalanges in the thumb joint and three in each finger.

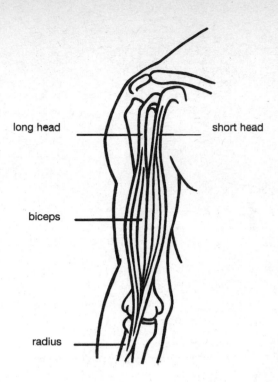

long head — short head

biceps

radius

biceps brachii

Muscles of the arm

Anterior flexor group
1 The **biceps brachii** (biceps=two heads of origin, brachion=arm) is a two-headed muscle situated at the front of the upper arm.

    Origin – by two heads from the scapula
    Insertion – radius and the deep fascia of the forearm
    Function – flexion of the elbow joint, supination (turning the palm upwards) of the forearm

The biceps are used powerfully when lifting or throwing any heavy weights, in racket sports and also supinating movements such as screwing in screws.

2 The **coracobrachialis** (caraco=coracoid process) is found in the upper part of the arm

Origin – scapula (coracoid process)
Insertion – humerus (middle third)
Function – flexion of the arm

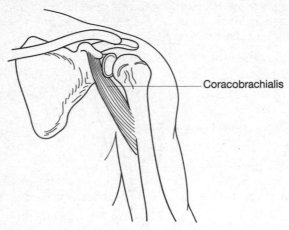

coracobrachialis

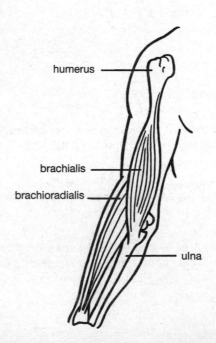

3 The **brachialis** is situated at the front of the upper arm and lies deep to the biceps.

Origin – humerus
Insertion – ulna
Function – flexion of the elbow

Where there are problems with this muscle, pains and pins and needles may be referred to the hands especially on the thumb side due to entrapment of the radial nerve.

4 The **brachioradialis** (radialis=radius)

Origin – humerus
Insertion – radius
Function – flexion of the elbow

Pain can radiate from this muscle down into the radial side (thumb side) of the wrist.

Posterior extensor group
The **triceps brachii** (triceps=three heads of origin) is the only muscle found on the back of the upper arm and it has three parts.

Origin – scapula (long head) and humerus (medial and lateral heads)
Insertion – ulna just below the elbow
Function – extension of the elbow joint

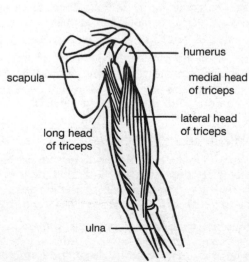

triceps brachii

The triceps muscle is the strongest muscle in the arm. Pain arising from the triceps muscle is often felt on the inside of the elbow joint. It is put under strain when lifting or throwing heavy weights.

Supination (turning the palm upwards) is performed by the **supinator** muscle as well as by the biceps brachii.

Pronation (turning the palm downwards) is performed by the **pronator teres** and the **pronator quadratus**.

Muscles moving the wrist and fingers
There is a large number of muscles moving the hands and fingers.

The anterior group of muscles function as flexors.

The posterior group of muscles function as extensors.

Flexors of the wrist
These include the **flexor carpi radialis, flexor carpi ulnaris** and the **palmaris longus**.

Origin – humerus (medial epicondyle) – this is the bump on the inside at the bottom of the humerus (little finger side)
Insertion – carpals, metacarpals and phalanges
Function – flexion of the wrist (bending the wrist up towards the body with the palm upwards)

Extensors of the wrist
These include **extensor carpi radialis longus, extensor carpi radialis brevis** and the **extensor carpi ulnaris**.

Origin – humerus (lateral epicondyle) – this is the bump on the outside at the bottom of the humerus (thumb side)
Insertion – carpals, metacarpals and phalanges
Function – extension of the wrist (bending the wrist up towards the body with the palm downwards)

Muscles moving the fingers

The flexor muscles include the **flexor digitorum profundus** (deep flexor muscle of the fingers) and the **flexor digitorum superficialis** (surface flexor muscle of the fingers), which not only flex the fingers but also assist with flexion of the wrist.

Extensor muscles include the **extensor digitorum** (extensor muscle of the fingers) arising from the common extensor tendon attachment on the lateral epicondyle of the humerus inserting into the fingers. This muscle extends the fingers and also assists extension of the wrist. The **extensor indicis** (extensor muscle of the index finger) arises from the lower part of the ulna and extends the index finger. Finally the **extensor digiti minimi** arising from the common extensor tendon extends the little finger.

The main problem affecting the forearm muscles is overstrain injuries. Occupations such as typing, which involve repetitive movements, hobbies such as gardening and knitting and racket sports such as tennis and golf can give rise to problems and intense pain in the elbow joint. Pain may be referred to the wrist and fingers and may even radiate into the shoulders.

MUSCLES OF THE LOWER ARM

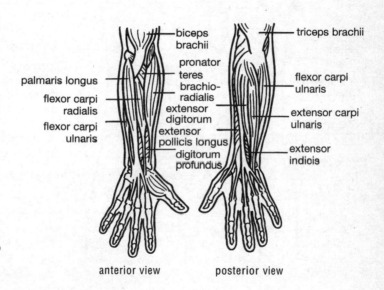

anterior view   posterior view

The abdomen

The colon is divided into the following portions: ascending, transverse, descending and sigmoid. The ascending colon lies in the vertical position on the right side of the abdomen. The transverse colon passes horizontally across the abdomen below the liver, stomach and spleen. It extends from the hepatic flexure to the splenic flexure. The descending colon is situated in the vertical position on the left-hand side of the abdomen. The sigmoid colon continues on downwards to become the rectum which terminates in the anal canal.

Muscles of the abdomen
Anterior and lateral parts of the abdominal wall

Four pairs of muscles, arranged in four layers form the lateral and anterior parts of the abdominal wall.

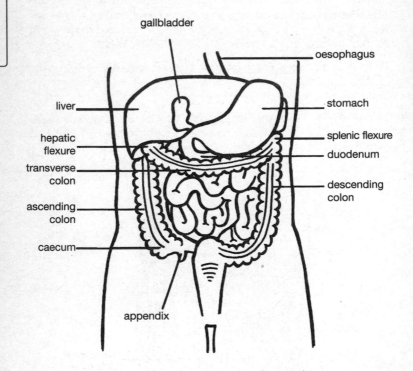

gallbladder

oesophagus

liver

stomach

hepatic flexure

splenic flexure

transverse colon

duodenum

ascending colon

descending colon

caecum

appendix

the digestive system

1 The **rectus abdominis** (rectus=fibres parallel to the midline, abdominois=abdomen) is the most superficial muscle of the abdominal wall. It is a broad flat muscle.

Origin – pubic bone and symphysis pubis
Insertion – lower ribs and sternum
Function – flexion of the trunk (forward bending as in sit-ups)

2 The **external oblique** (oblique = fibres diagonal to midline)

Origin – lower ribs
Insertion – iliac crest
Function – side bends the trunk (contraction of one side), compresses the abdomen (contraction of both sides)

3 The **internal oblique** lies deep to the external oblique.

Origin – crest of the ilium and the lumbar vertebrae
Insertion – lower ribs
The fibres of the internal oblique run at right angles to those of the external oblique
Function – same as the external oblique

4 The **transversus abdominis** (transverse=fibres perpendicular to the midline) is the deepest muscle of the abdominal wall. The fibres lie at right angles to the rectus abdominis.

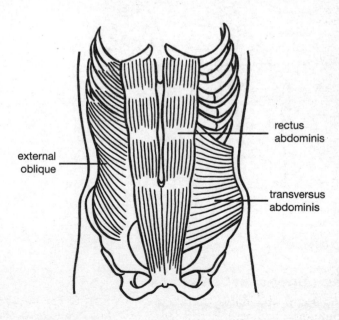

external
oblique

rectus
abdominis

transversus
abdominis

abdominal muscles

Origin – iliac crest and lumbar vertebrae
Insertion – the linea alba (this is a strong tendinous cord which extends from the sternum to the symphysis pubis. It looks like a seam running up the middle of the abdomen – in pregnancy it becomes pigmented)
Function – compresses the abdomen

The muscles forming the posterior part of the abdominal wall are the **internal oblique, transversus abdominis, quadratus lumborum** and the **psoas.**

The **Iliopsoas** (psoa=muscle of the loin)

Together the psoas major and the iliacus are termed the iliopoas.

Origin – front of the lumbar vertebrae
Insertion – femur (inside top)
Function – flexion and lateral rotation (turning outwards of the hip); flexion of the spine

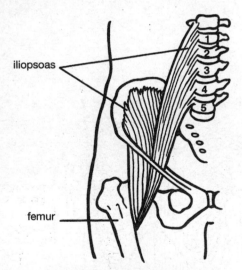

iliopsoas

The upper chest and neck

Muscles of the chest and neck

1 The **pectoralis major** is the main muscle of the chest area.

Origin – clavicle, sternum and upper ribs
Insertion – top of the humerus

Function – medial rotation (inward rotation) of the arm – i.e. draws the arm across the chest; adduction of the arm

Tightness in the **pectoral** muscles gives rise to sensitivity in the chest area and when it appears on the left-hand side it may simulate and create fears of coronary disease. Any chest pain should obviously be examined by a medical practitioner.

Other muscles of the chest include the **pectoralis minor** which lies underneath the pectoralis minor and the **subclavius** muscle.

2 The **sternocleidomastoid** (sternum=breastbone, cleido= clavicle, mastoid-mastoid process of temporal bone of the skull) is one of the principal and largest neck muscles.

Origin – sternum and clavicle
Insertion – temporal bone (mastoid process) – i.e. behind the ear at the back of the head
Function – contraction of both sides causes flexion of the head (bending the head forward); contraction of one side allows turning of the head from side to side and also inclination of the head towards the shoulder.

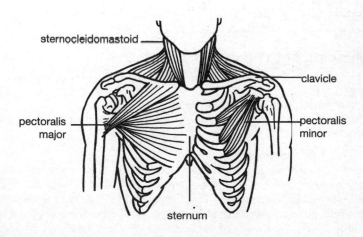

chest and neck muscles

If this muscle goes into spasm the condition is called 'wryneck' or 'torticollis'.

3 The **splenius capitis** (splenion=bandage) is the bandage shaped muscle of the neck.

> Origin: The seventh cervical vertebrae and the upper three or four thoracic vertebrae
> Insertion: The mastoid process of the temporal bone
> Function: Extends and rotates the head

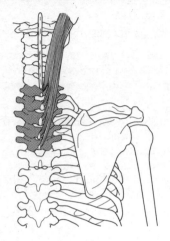

splenius capitis

Muscles of the head and face

The following muscles are the main muscles of the head and face.

Muscles of facial expression

These muscles are responsible for a remarkable range of facial expressions.

1 The occipitofrontalis

Position – the occipitalis and the frontalis are collectively known as the occipitofrontalis. This muscle is also known as the epicranius. The occipitalis (epicranial frontal belly) is a muscle sheath extending over the back of the skull (the occipital bone). The frontalis is a sheath of muscle over the front of the skull (the frontal and parietal bones). Together they cover the skull rather like a cap.

Function – occipitalis draws the scalp backwards; frontalis – moves the scalp forwards (wrinkles the forehead horizontally) and raises the eyebrows.

2 The corrugator supercilii
Position – the corrugator muscles are small muscles located between the frontal bone and the skin of the eyebrows.

Function – they draw the eyebrows down and towards each other, i.e. they wrinkle the forehead vertically to produce a frown (*corrugo* means to wrinkle).

3 The procerus
Position – the small procerus muscles are found on the nasal bones.

Function – they wrinkle the nose to create an expression of disgust!

4 The orbicularis oculi
Position – the orbicularis oculi muscles encircle the eyes.

Function – they close the eyes. If you wink or blink these muscles are used.

5 The nasalis
Position – the nasalis muscles cross over the bridge of the nose.

Function – they dilate (open up) the nostrils and would be used when flaring the nostrils!

6 The levator labii superioris
Position – these are thin bands of muscles running from under the eye to the mouth.

Function – they raise the upper lip producing a cheerful expression.

7 The zygomaticus (minor and major)
Position – this thin muscle pair extend diagonally from the zygomatic bones to the angle of the mouth (major) and to the upper lip (minor). They are superficial to the masseter muscles.

Function – they draw the angle of the mouth upward and backward as in laughing.

8 The levator anguli oris
Position – these thin bands of muscle run from the maxilla to the corner of the mouth. They lie below the levator labii superioris.

Function – they raise the corner of the mouth producing a cheerful expression.

9 The buccinator
Position – these are the major muscles of the cheek lying deep to the masseter muscles (*bucc* means cheek).

Function – they are used for whistling and also blowing as when playing a trumpet. The buccinator muscles also draw the cheeks in towards the teeth as when chewing.

10 The **risorius**
Position – the risorius muscles run towards the corners of the mouth.

Function – they retract the angle of the mouth as when grinning (*risor* means laughter).

11 The **orbicularis oris**
Position – the orbicularis oris encircles the mouth.

Function – it closes and protrudes the lips as in kissing.

12 The **depressor anguli oris (triangularis)**
Position – these muscles extend from the mandible to the corners of the mouth.

Function – they pull down the corners of the mouth as when frowning.

13 The **depressor labii inferioris**
Position – these muscles are located between the mandible (mid-chin) and skin of the lower lip.

Function – they draw the lower lip downwards to create a sulky expression.

14 The **mentalis**
Position – the mentalis muscles form a V-shape over the centre of the chin.

Function – they raise and protrude the lower lip and also wrinkle the skin of the chin.

15 The **platysma**
Position – the platysma is a superficial broad sheet-like muscle extending from the upper fourth of the chest up the sides of the neck to the chin, jaw and mandible.

Function – it depresses the lower lip and also draws up the skin of the chest. The platysma muscle is used when yawning.

Muscles of mastication

The following muscles are responsible for chewing.

1 The **temporalis**
Position – the fan-shaped temporalis muscles are at the side of the head and extend from the temporal bone in front and above the ear down to the lower jaw.

Function – they close the lower jaw, clench the teeth and help with the chewing action.

2 The **masseter**
Position – the masseter muscles extend from the cheekbone to the mandible.

Function – they close the lower jaw and clench the teeth (*master* means chewer).

3 The **pterygoids (medial and lateral)**
Position – the pterygoids are deep muscles which act on the jaw.

Function – the medial pterygoid closes the lower jaw and clenches the teeth. The lateral pterygoid opens the jaw, protrudes the mandible and moves the mandible from side to side.

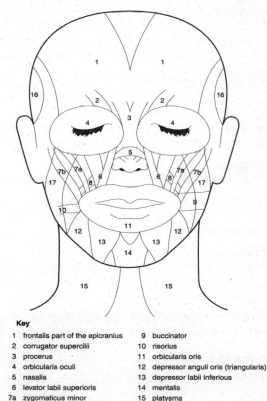

Key

1	frontalis part of the epicranius	9	buccinator
2	corrugator supercilii	10	risorius
3	procerus	11	orbicularis oris
4	orbicularis oculi	12	depressor anguli oris (triangularis)
5	nasalis	13	depressor labii inferious
6	levator labii superioris	14	mentalis
7a	zygomaticus minor	15	platysma
7b	zygomaticus major	16	temporalis
8	levator anguli oris	17	masseter

muscles of facial expression and mastication

Further reading

Anthony and Thibodeau *Textbook of Anatomy and Physiology*, Mosby, 1983

Brown D. *Teach Yourself Hand Reflexology*, Hodder & Stoughton, 2003

Brown D. *Yeach Yourself Indian Head Massage*, Hodder & Stoughton, 2003

Brown D. *Teach Yourself Aromatherapy*, Hodder & Stoughton, 1996

Diamond H. and M. *Fit for Life*, London, Bantam Press, 1987

Doyle, Wendy *Teach Yourself Healthy Eating*, Hodder & Stoughton, 1994

Grisogno, Vivian *Sports Injuries*, London, John Murray, 1984

Grant, D. and Joice J. *Food Combining for Health*, London, Thorsons, 1984

Kenton, L. *Raw Energy*, London, Century, 1984

Leboyer, F. *Loving Hands*, Collins, 1977

Peterson, Lars and Per Renstrom *Sports Injuries*, London, Dunitz, 1984

Tortora and Anagnostakos *Principles of Anatomy & Physiology*, Harper and Row, 1984

Valnet Dr J. *The Practice of Aromatherapy*, C.W. Daniel, 1982

Walker Dr N. W. *Diet and Salad*, Norwalk Press, 1971

Useful addresses

UK

Beaumont College of Natural Medicine
MWB Business Exchange
23 Hinton Road, Bournemouth, BH1 2EF
Tel: +44 (0)1202 708887
www.beaumontcollege.co.uk
Information on professional training courses under the personal direction of Denise Whichello Brown

Denise Brown Essential Oils
Tel: +44 (0)1202 708887
www.denisebrown.co.uk
For a wide selection of high quality pure unadulterated essential oils, base oils, creams and lotions, relaxation music, wall charts etc. (International Mail Order)

Osteopathic Centre for Children
109 Harley Street, London W1G 6AN
Tel: +44 (0)20 7486 6160
www.occ.uk.com

The Association of Osteomyologists (Manual Therapy)
80 Greenstead Avenue, Woodford Green, Essex IG8 7ER
Tel: +44 (0)20 8504 1462
www.osteomyology.co.uk

The Society of Homeopaths
4a Artizan Road, Northampton NN1 4HU
Tel: +44 (0)1604 621400
www.homeopathy-soh.org
The largest organization registering professional homoeopaths
in the UK

British Homeopathic Association
15 Clerkenwell Close, London EC1R 0AA
Tel: +44 (0)20 7566 7800
www.trusthomeopathy.org
Helpful information about homeopathy

Integral Yoga
293 Malmesbury Park Road
Charminster, Bournemouth BH8 8PX
Tel: +44 (0)1202 251548
Offers a wide range of classes.

US

www.aboutmassage.com
A site that has information on massage associations based in the
USA

American Academy of Osteopathy
www.academyofosteopathy.org
Tel: +1 (317) 879-1881

index

teach yourself®

Hinduism
History, 101 Key Ideas
How to Win at Horse Racing
How to Win at Poker
HTML Publishing on the WWW
Human Anatomy & Physiology
Hungarian
Icelandic
Indian Head Massage
Indonesian
Information Technology, 101 Key Ideas
Internet, The
Irish
Islam
Italian
Italian, Beginner's
Italian Grammar
Italian Grammar, Quick Fix
Italian, Instant
Italian, Improve your
Italian Language, Life & Culture
Italian Verbs
Italian Vocabulary
Japanese
Japanese, Beginner's
Japanese, Instant
Japanese Language, Life & Culture
Japanese Script, Beginner's
Java
Jewellery Making
Judaism
Korean
Latin
Latin American Spanish
Latin, Beginner's
Latin Dictionary
Latin Grammar
Letter Writing Skills
Linguistics
Linguistics, 101 Key Ideas
Literature, 101 Key Ideas
Mahjong
Managing Stress
Marketing
Massage
Mathematics
Mathematics, Basic
Media Studies
Meditation
Mosaics
Music Theory
Needlecraft
Negotiating
Nepali

Norwegian
Origami
Panjabi
Persian, Modern
Philosophy
Philosophy of Mind
Philosophy of Religion
Philosophy of Science
Philosophy, 101 Key Ideas
Photography
Photoshop
Physics
Piano
Planets
Planning Your Wedding
Polish
Politics
Portuguese
Portuguese, Beginner's
Portuguese Grammar
Portuguese, Instant
Portuguese Language, Life & Culture
Postmodernism
Pottery
Powerpoint 2002
Presenting for Professionals
Project Management
Psychology
Psychology, 101 Key Ideas
Psychology, Applied
Quark Xpress
Quilting
Recruitment
Reflexology
Reiki
Relaxation
Retaining Staff
Romanian
Russian
Russian, Beginner's
Russian Grammar
Russian, Instant
Russian Language, Life & Culture
Russian Script, Beginner's
Sanskrit
Screenwriting
Serbian
Setting up a Small Business
Shorthand, Pitman 2000
Sikhism
Spanish
Spanish, Beginner's
Spanish Grammar
Spanish Grammar, Quick Fix

Spanish, Instant
Spanish, Improve your
Spanish Language, Life & Culture
Spanish Starter Kit
Spanish Verbs
Spanish Vocabulary
Speaking on Special Occasions
Speed Reading
Statistical Research
Statistics
Swahili
Swahili Dictionary
Swedish
Tagalog
Tai Chi
Tantric Sex
Teaching English as a Foreign Language
Teaching English One to One
Teams and Team-Working
Thai
Time Management
Tracing your Family History
Travel Writing
Trigonometry
Turkish
Turkish, Beginner's
Typing
Ukrainian
Urdu
Urdu Script, Beginner's
Vietnamese
Volcanoes
Watercolour Painting
Weight Control through Diet and
  Exercise
Welsh
Welsh Dictionary
Welsh Language, Life & Culture
Wills and Probate
Wine Tasting
Winning at Job Interviews
Word 2002
World Faiths
Writing a Novel
Writing for Children
Writing Poetry
Xhosa
Yoga
Zen
Zulu

teach
yourself

Indian head massage
denise whichello brown

- Do you want to know more about this ancient therapy?
- Do you want to understand the basic principles?
- Are you looking for a therapy you can apply to your own life?

Indian Head Massage is a comprehensive introduction to this ancient holistic therapy that balances body, mind and spirit to promote health and well-being. The book explains the origins and benefits of Indian head massage and its basic techniques and gives clear, step-by-step instructions and advice on the best oils to use. Use the quick-and-easy treatments on yourself or you friends and family, anytime, anywhere, to improve your health and well-being.

Denise Whichello Brown is a highly acclaimed practitioner, lecturer and author of international repute, with over 20 years' experience in complementary medicine.

teach
yourself

aromatherapy
denise whichello brown

- Do you want to understand the principles of aromatherapy?
- Are you confused by the different oils and techniques?
- Do you need to help in finding the remedy which is right for you?

Aromatherapy is a complete guide to this ancient and popular
technique. It gives you clear and detailed information on the
physical, emotional and spiritual effects of 40 essential oils and
explains the various techniques for using them safely and
effectively in all areas of your life, including for pregnancy and
childbirth and with babies and children.

Denise Whichello Brown is a highly acclaimed practitioner,
lecturer and author of international repute, with over 20 years'
experience in complementary medicine.

teach
yourself

hand reflexology
denise whichello brown

- Do you want to discover an ideal way of treating yourself?
- Are you looking for an easy-to-follow guide to basic hand reflexology techniques?
- Do you want to know how to treat and eliminate many common medical problems?

Hand Reflexology is a simple, straightforward and practical guide to this ancient and increasingly popular healing art. Discover how reflexology has an enormous part to play in healthcare and how it offers much more than just a hand massage. Explore the roots of reflexology, and learn techniques easily with step-by-step instructions with accompanying illustrations.

Denise Whichello Brown is a highly acclaimed practitioner, lecturer and author of international repute, with over 20 years' experience in complementary medicine.